Renal Diet CookBook

Food Recipes for Kidney Disease and Dialysis

Joanna Aphiah

Renal Diet CookBook: **Food Recipes for Kidney Disease & Dialysis** by Joanna Aphiah.

Published by Kwizbud Publishing House, 204C Chestnut Crossing Dr.,Newark 19713, New Jersey, U.S.A.

Books@kwizbud.com

ISBN: 9781675586778

Table of Contents

PREFACE

Renal failure is the inability of the kidney to perform its functions. Major risk factors include high blood pressure, diabetes, a family history of kidney failure, and being age 60 or older. This leaves the victims in a complete state of grief as they move from bad to terrible.

With the onset of renal failure, it is expedient that your diet immediately changes to accommodate the inability of your kidney to process certain nutrients in our regular foods.

Renal Diet Cookbook: Food Recipes for Kidney Disease and Dialysis provides precise information that anyone in this condition needs. While I advise and expect you are already consulting a dietician, this book helps you process all the numerous information that is hitting you at the moment.

You will be well again. I am in no doubt that your health will be significantly restored as you implement the diet guidance in this cookbook along with your dietician and physician..

Joanna Aphiah

This is not just a recipe book. Joanna has set out to educate patients, care-givers and her readers in general about kidney disease, explaining why adopting a healthy diet is important. I also find the included meal plan, very essential.

- *Soso Harcourt, MD, President*
Caritas Kidney Centre

1.0 Introduction
What Does "Renal Diet" Mean?

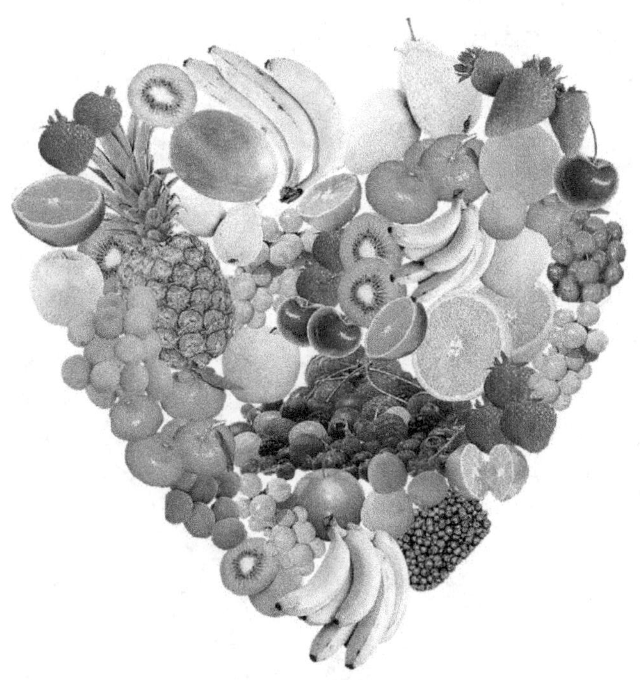

A renal diet is a healthy way of caring for your kidney and gut environment. When you have a healthy gut, it serves as the primary protection for your kidney. One of the best ways this can be achieved is to eat plant-based diets made up of fiber and probiotic foods. Each individual is different, so also the gut microbe. There are, however, standards, and according to medical experts, certain types of food tend to resonate well and keep our kidney safe. There are, however, others we should avoid.

2.0

Facts about

Renal Diet

2.1 Take Less Potassium, Less Phosphorus and Less Sodium

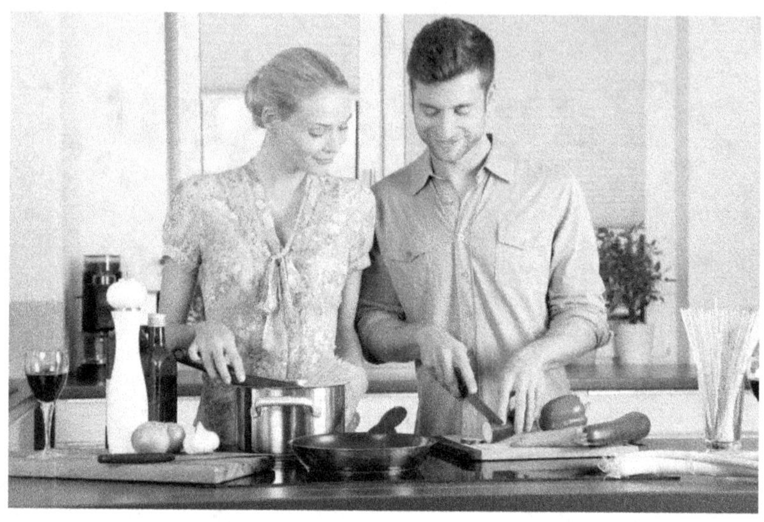

Consume less salt and fewer salty foods. In doing this, you will be controlling your blood pressure and helping dialysis during kidney failure.

- Try using herbs, spices, and low-salt flavor boosters as a salt replacement

- Again, try to avoid potassium made foods.

2.2 How Can I Meet My Protein Needs?

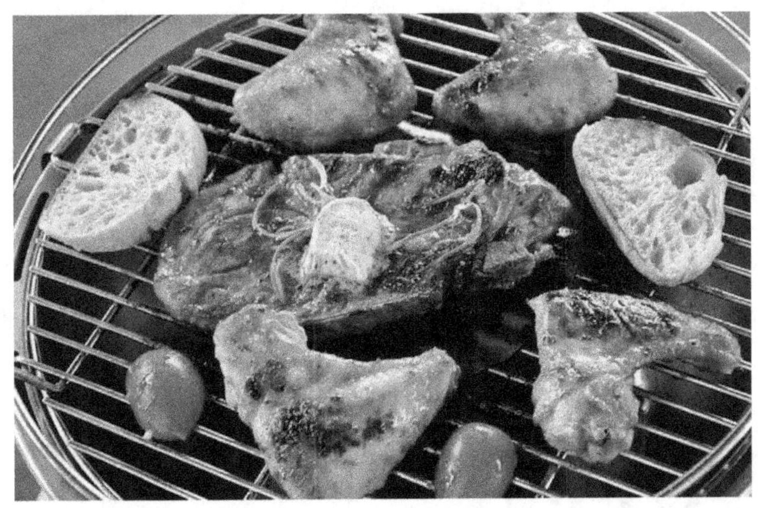

There is a need to eat more protein, especially when you are on dialysis. It strengthens and builds up the body system. High protein food (meat, fish, poultry, fresh pork, or eggs)

repairs tissues and significantly improve health when eaten at least 9 ounces each day.

You can combine with pork chop, chicken breast, and butter.

Note: there is lesser protein in the following foods: peanut butter, nuts, seeds, dried beans, peas, and lentils.

You are allowed to eat from animal proteins like beef, lamb, pork, and poultry. Fish are very rich in protein. Eat them to get the required quantity each day.

If there is any instance where you shouldn't eat meats for protein, take little amounts of fish per day, and also you can mix it with the following dishes such as in soups, salads, pasta, sandwiches.

2.3 Grains and Cereals

Consume as many grains and cereals as you like. Only if you are involved in a weight loss program and watching your calorie intake should you limit its consumption. Grains, cereals, and slices of white bread are an excellent source of calories. You need **6 -11 servings from this group each day**.

2.4 Ten Foods You Must Avoid In Your Renal Diet

- Potatoes (including French Fries, potato chips and sweet potatoes)

- Tomatoes and tomato sauce

- Winter squash

- Pumpkin

- Asparagus (cooked)

- Avocado

- Beets

- Beet greens

- Cooked spinach

- Parsnips and rutabaga

2.5 Ten Essential Foods for Renal Diet

If you have been diagnosed of kidney disease then it is recommended that you discuss your daily meals with your dietician. Here are ten essential foods that have proven capability to improve the health of your kidney:

1. Red bell peppers as a vegetable is an ideal kidney diet because of its low potassium content. Besides being a

nice source of vitamins A, C, and B6; Red bell peppers are also a major source of lycopene, which is a well known antioxidant that protects the body against certain cancers.

2. Cabbage is high in vitamin C, vitamin K, vitamin B6, folic acid and fiber, cabbage is also low in potassium. Raw cabbage makes a fantastic addition to the dialysis diet as topping for fish tacos or as coleslaw.

3. Cauliflower is a cruciferous vegetable known to be rich in vitamin C and a good source of fiber and folate. It contains glucosinolates, indoles, and thiocyanates, which help the liver fight off toxins. These toxins are substances that could potentially damage cell membranes and DNA. It can be consumed steamed, raw, or in

soups. Steam and mash to use as an alternative to mashed Cauliflower.

4. Garlic: Is a herb that is healthy when consumed in food. However, in pill form, it can alter liver enzymes, thin the blood, and change kidney functions. That said, recent evidence suggest that garlic is beneficial in promoting overall kidney health due to its diuretic properties

5. Onions: is a powerful antioxidant that is known for being low in potassium and rich in flavonoids, especially quercetin, that works to reduce heart disease and protects against most cancers. Onions are a good source of chromium that helps with carbohydrate, fat, and protein metabolism.

6. Apples are known to help reduce cholesterol, protect against heart disease, prevent constipation, and reduce cancer risk. Apples also contain anti-inflammatory compounds, and like it is said, än apple a day will keep the doctor away.

7. Cherries are rich in phytochemicals and antioxidants and have been shown that Gout patients who eat cherries usually lower their risk of gout attacks and inflammation when eaten daily. Note that kidney disease causes gout; yet gout might also lead to kidney disease.

8. Red grapes contain vitamin C and several flavonoids, which give it its characteristic red color and known to reduce inflammation. Red grapes

are also high in resveratrol, that has been shown to improve heart health while protecting against diabetes and cognitive decline

9. Ginger also contains vitamin B5, manganese, and magnesium. The rhizome of the ginger plant is a rich source of antioxidants, including zingerones, gingerols, shogaols, and other ketone derivatives, making it a great addition to any diet. Ginger has sedative, analgesic, antibacterial, and antipyretic properties. Ginger may prevent diabetic kidney damage, joint pain and also reduces nausea

10. Coriander is a herb with a pleasant flavor and aroma, making it an excellent addition to many food dishes. Coriander is a good source of

vitamins B2, A, K, and C. It is also rich in calcium, selenium, iron, manganese, and fiber.

2.6: How a Serving Goes

- 1 slice bread (white, rye, or sourdough)

- ½ English muffin

- ½ bagel

- ½ hamburger bun

- ½ hot dog bun

- 1 6-inch tortilla

- ½ cup cooked pasta

- ½ cup cooked white rice

- ½ cup cooked cereal (like cream of wheat)

- 1 cup cold cereal (like corn flakes or crispy rice)

- 4 unsalted crackers

- 1½ cups unsalted popcorn

- 10 vanilla wafers

Fruits:

- Apple (1)

- Berries (½ cup)

- Cherries (10)

- Fruit cocktail, drained (½ cup)

- Grapes (15)

- Peach (1 small fresh or canned, drained)

- Pear, fresh or canned, drained (1 halve)

- Pineapple (½ cup canned, drained)

- Plums (1-2)

- Tangerine (1)

- Watermelon (1 small wedge)

Drinks:

- Apple cider

- Cranberry juice cocktail

- Grape juice

- Lemonade

Vegetables/Salads :

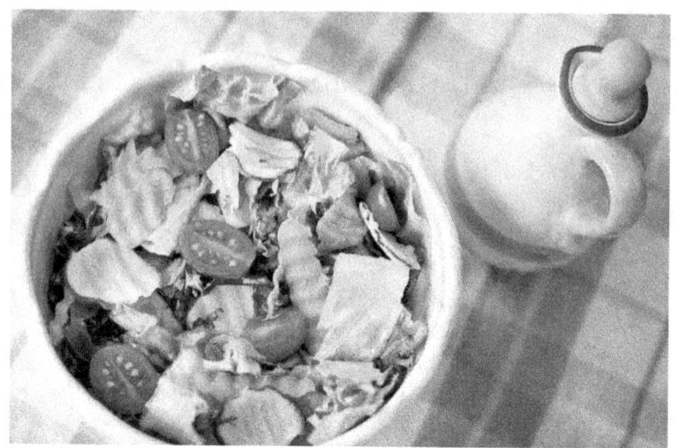

When you limit the consumption of certain vegetables, you help keep your heart under control.

Eat 2-3 servings of these low-potassium vegetables every day. One serving = ½-cup.

Choose:

- Broccoli (raw or cooked from frozen)

- Cabbage

- Carrots

- Cauliflower

- Celery

- Cucumber

- Eggplant

- Garlic

- Green and Wax beans ("string beans")

- Lettuce-all types (1 cup)

- Onion

- Peppers-all types and colors

- Radishes

- Watercress

- Zucchini and Yellow squash

3.0
Healthy Renal
Diet Recipes

3.1 Important Facts

The following are foods you should eat at various stages of kidney disease. Dairy and small amounts of protein including eggs, poultry, pork, and beef. Vegetables that are small or medium in potassium like eggplant, bean sprouts, lettuce, celery, and asparagus. Starches such as pasta, bread, popcorn, cereal, rice, and unsalted crackers. Fruits with small to medium potassium content like pears, grapes, blueberries, peaches, and mangoes.

Fats like margarine, butter, or oil should be limited to about one tablespoon a day. However your doctor will have the final say on which foods you should eat while on treatment for kidney failure.

Chili Rice with Beef

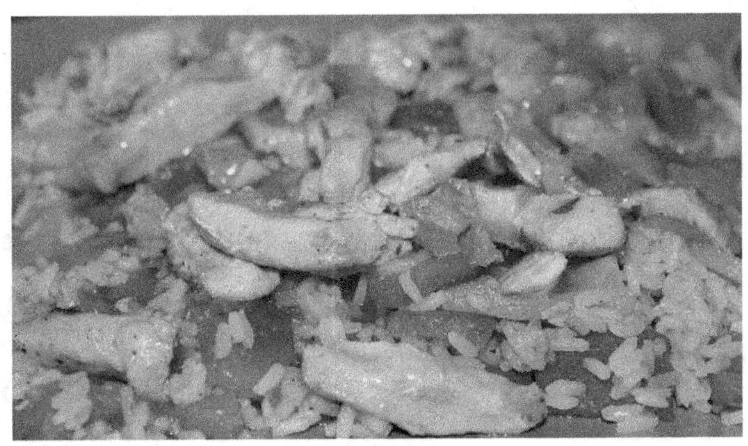

Ingredients

2 tablespoons olive oil

1 pound lean ground beef

1 cup onion, chopped

2 cups rice, cooked

1 ½ teaspoons chili con carne seasoning powder

⅛ teaspoon black pepper

½ teaspoon sage

Preparation

1. Get a cooking pan and pour in some oil for heating. Chop your beef and add in some onions. Cook, occasionally stirring until browned.

2. Pour in the rice and seasonings. Use a spoon and mix together.

3. When done, take off from the heat and place in a bowl. Allow cooling for ten minutes before serving.

Nutritional Information

360 calories 1g trans fat 78 mg sodium

23g protein 65 mg cholesterol 427 mg potassium

14g total fat 26g carbohydrate 233 mg phosphorus

4g saturated fat 2g fiber 34 mg calcium

Yield: 4

Salisbury Steak

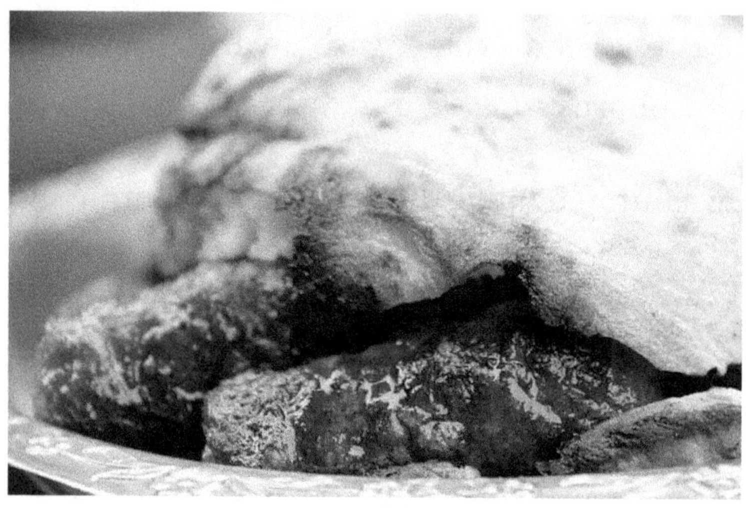

Ingredients

1 tablespoon corn starch

1 pound lean ground beef or chicken or turkey or chopped steak,

½ cup green pepper, chopped

1 small onion, chopped

1 teaspoon black pepper

1 egg

1 tablespoon olive oil

½ cup of water

Preparations

1. Combine the following ingredients in a big bowl: meat, onion, green pepper, black pepper, and egg. Form into patties.

2. Get a kitchen skillet, pour some oil and heat it up. Add the initial patties that were formed earlier. Flip and cook on both sides

3. Pour water up to half and cook for 15 minutes. Remove patties from heat.

4. To your drippings, add remaining water and corn starch. Cook on low heat and stirring continually, So it thickens.

5. Remove when done and pour gravy over steak.

Nutritional Information

249 calories 0g trans fat 128 mg sodium

22g protein 149 mg cholesterol 366 mg potassium

57g total fat 7g carbohydrate 218 mg phosphorus

3g saturated fat 1gram fiber 33 mg calcium

Yield: 4

Parsley Burger

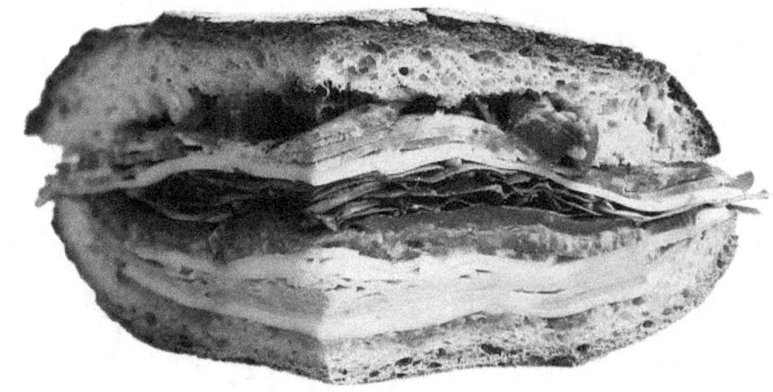

Ingredients

¼ teaspoon oregano

1 pound ground turkey or ground lean meat

1 tablespoon parsley flakes

¼ teaspoon black pepper

¼ teaspoon ground thyme

1 tablespoon lemon juice

Preparations

1. Combine your ingredients thoroughly.

2. Scoop and make into four small patties about ¾" thick.

3. pour grease on a skillet and place the patties on it.

4. Broil about 3"-4" from the heat for 10-15 minutes, stirring occasionally.

Nutritional Information

171 calories 0g trans fat 108 mg sodium

20g protein 90 mg cholesterol 289 mg potassium

10g total fat 0g   carbohydrate 180 mg phosphorus

3g saturated fat 0g fiber 21 mg calcium

Yield: 4

Swedish Meatballs

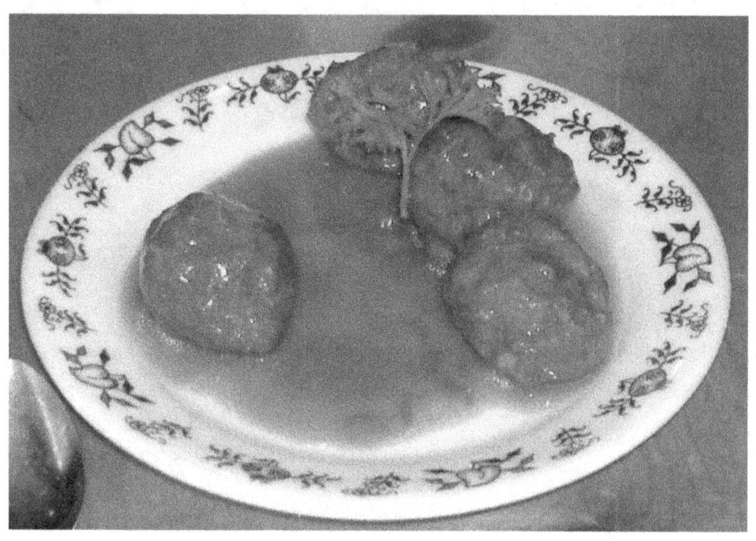

Ingredients for sauce

¼ cup of olive oil

2 tablespoons all-purpose flour

1 teaspoon onion powder

2 teaspoons vinegar

2 teaspoons stevia

1 teaspoon Tabasco sauce

2-3 cups water

Preparations for sauce

1. Get a saucepan and mix oil and flour in it. Cook and fry until brown then remove from heat.

2. Add the following; onion powder, vinegar, stevia, Tabasco sauce, and water.

3. Restore heat, and keep stirring until thickened.

Yield: 35

Ingredients for meatballs

Serving size: 2 meatballs

1 pound lean ground beef or turkey

¼ cup of onions, finely chopped

1 tablespoon lemon juice

1 teaspoon poultry seasoning (without salt)

1 teaspoon black pepper

¼ teaspoon dry mustard

¾ teaspoon onion powder

1 teaspoon Italian seasoning

1 teaspoon granulated stevia

1 teaspoon Tabasco sauce

Preparing meatballs

1. Preheat your oven to 425°F.

2. Combine all ingredients well.

3. Scoop meatballs with a tablespoon meat mixture for each meatball.

4. Get a dish and place your meatballs in it. Next, you bake for 20 minutes.

5. Transfer your fried meatballs from oven and add to sauce.

Nutritional Information

76 calories 0g trans fat 31 mg sodium

5g protein 21 mg cholesterol 70-milligram potassium

6g total fat 2g carbohydrate 44 mg phosphorus

1g saturated fat 0g fiber 7 mg calcium

Steak and Onion Sandwich

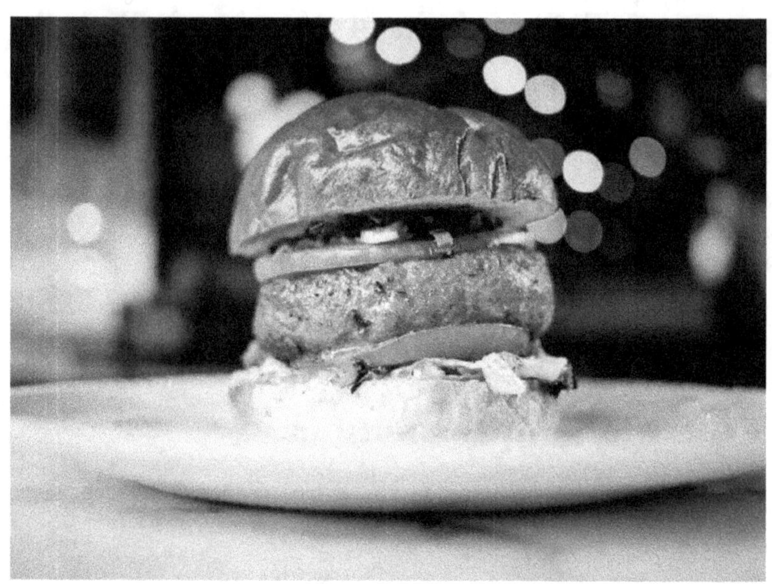

Ingredients

4 chopped steaks (4-ounces each)

1 tablespoon lemon juice

1 tablespoon Italian seasoning

1 tablespoon black pepper

1 tablespoon olive oil

1 medium onion, sliced into rings

4 hoagie rolls, sliced

Preparations

1. Mix the following ingredient first; meat with lemon juice, Italian seasoning and black pepper.

2. Get a kitchen pan, pour in some oil and heat over medium heat.

3. Pour in your steaks and cook until Brown. Flip both sides Remove and drain on paper towels.

4. Reduce heat; toss in onions and sauté until onions are soft.

5. Serve and garnish with onion rings.

Nutritional Information

345 calories 0g trans fat 247 mg sodium

14g protein 40 mg cholesterol 200 mg potassium

21g total fat 26g   carbohydrate 115 mg phosphorus

7g saturated fat 2g fiber 98 mg calcium

Taco Stuffing

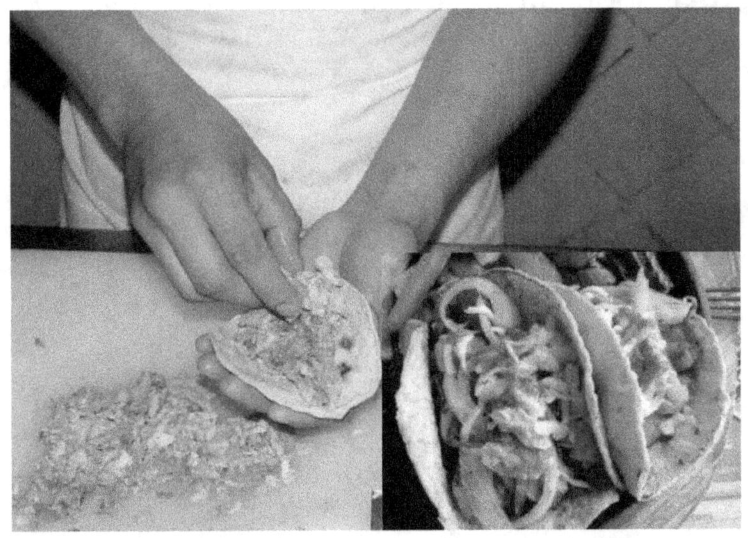

Ingredients

2 tablespoon olive oil

1 ¼ pounds lean ground beef or turkey

½ teaspoon ground red pepper

½ teaspoon black pepper

1 teaspoon Italian seasoning

1 teaspoon garlic powder

1 teaspoon onion powder

½ teaspoon Tabasco® sauce

½ teaspoon nutmeg

1 medium taco shells

½ head shredded lettuce

Preparations

1. Set a cooking pan and pour some oil in it. Heat oil. Combine the ground meat and all remaining ingredients except taco shells

and lettuce. Cook until ingredients are well-blended and beef is done.

2. Stuff your taco shells with 2-ounces of meat and garnish with shredded lettuce.

Nutritional Information

176 calories 0g trans fat 124 mg sodium

14g protein 56 mg cholesterol 258 mg potassium

9g total fat 9gcarbohydrate 150 mg phosphorus

2g saturated fat 0g fiber 33 mg calcium

Yield: 8

Basic Meat Loaf

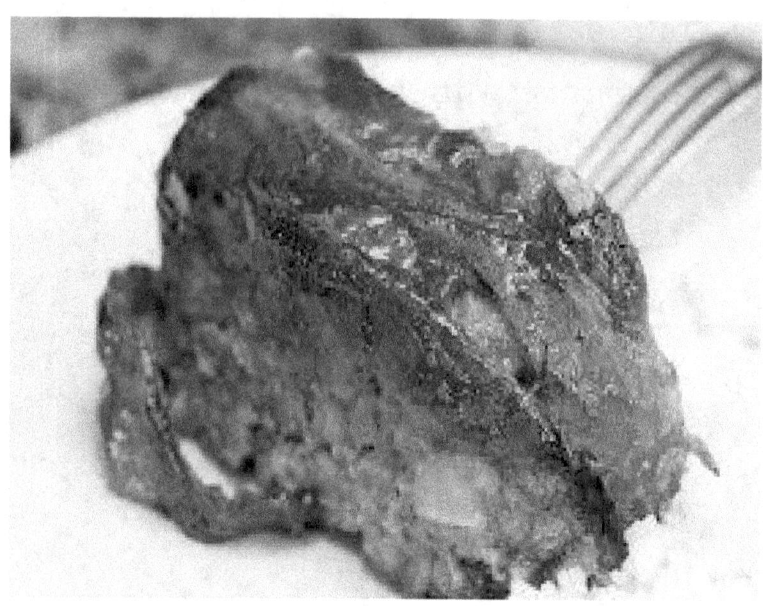

Ingredients

1 pound lean ground turkey

1 egg white

1 tablespoon lemon juice

½ cup plain bread crumbs

½ teaspoon onion powder

½ teaspoon Italian seasoning

¼ teaspoon black pepper

½ cup chopped onions

½ cup diced green bell pepper

¼ cup water

Preparations:

1. Preheat oven to 400°F.

2. Add some lemon juice over the meat.

3. Get a large bowl and mix remaining ingredients.

4. Add the ingredients to meat and mix well.

5. Put in a loaf pan; bake for 45 minutes.

Nutritional Information

110 calories 0g trans fat 71mg sodium

12g protein 42mg cholesterol 138mg potassium

5g total fat 2g carbohydrate 87 mg phosphorus

1g saturated fat 0g fiber 20mg calcium

Turkey and Noodles

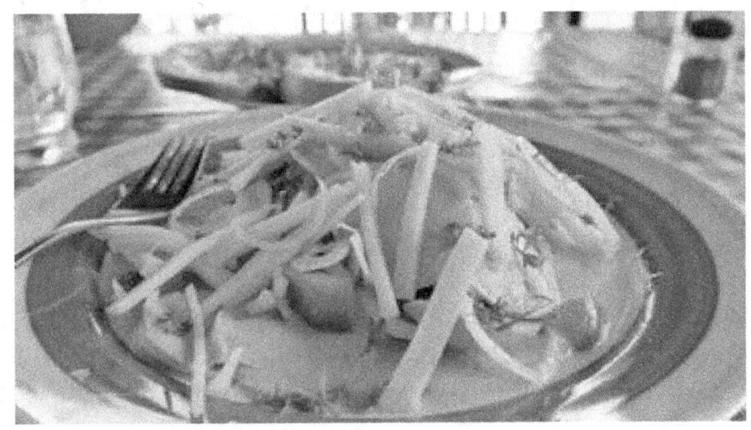

Ingredients

2 cups dry elbow macaroni

1 tablespoon olive or olive oil

2 pounds fresh lean ground turkey

½ cup green onions, chopped

½ cup green pepper, chopped

1 tablespoon Italian seasoning

1 teaspoon black pepper

Preparations

1. Cook macaroni with 4 cups of water in a medium boiler. Allow boiling for 5 minutes. Drain and set aside.

2. Pour in some oil and heat up in a large skillet over moderate heat. Pour in your ground turkey and cook until done, stirring occasionally.

3. Combine your onions, green peppers, Italian seasoning, black pepper, and cooked macaroni. Mix well.

4. Cover then cook with low heat for 5 minutes or until desired. Serve warm.

Nutritional Information

273 calories 0g trans fat 188 mg sodium

33g protein 80 mg cholesterol 533 mg potassium

7g total fat 22g carbohydrates 296 mg phosphorus

1g saturated fat 2g fiber 55 mg calcium

Yield: 8

Turkey Barbecue Cups

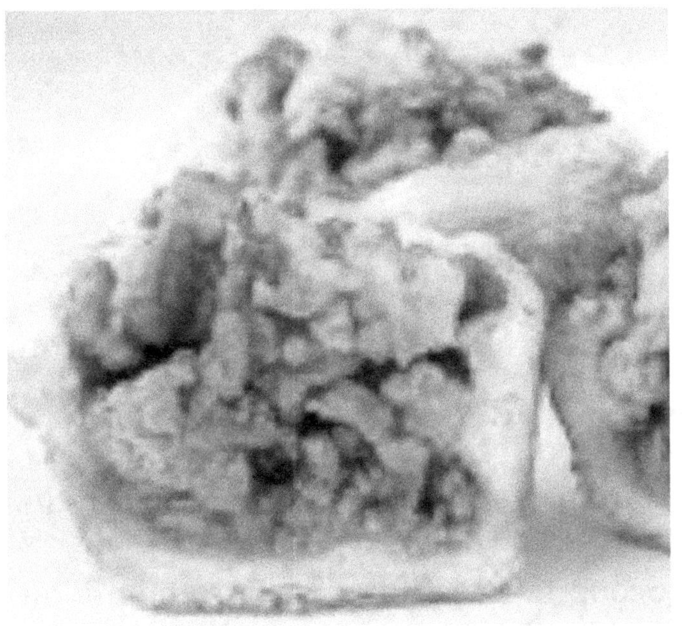

Ingredients

¾ pounds lean ground turkey

½ cup spicy barbecue sauce*

2 teaspoons onion flakes dash garlic powder

1 10-ounces package low-fat refrigerator biscuits

Preparations

1. Fry your turkey until brown.

2. Mix the following; barbecue sauce, onion flakes, and garlic powder.

3. Hard press each biscuit into a muffin tin.

4. Scoop the beef mixture into the middle of each biscuit cup.

5. Bake at 390°F for 12 to 15 minutes.

Nutritional Information

134 calories 0g trans fat 342 mg sodium

7g   protein 27 mg cholesterol 151 mg potassium

5g total fat 13g carbohydrate 152-milligram phosphorus

1g saturated fat 0g fiber 11 mg calcium

Yield: 10

Seafood Recipes

Seafood Croquettes

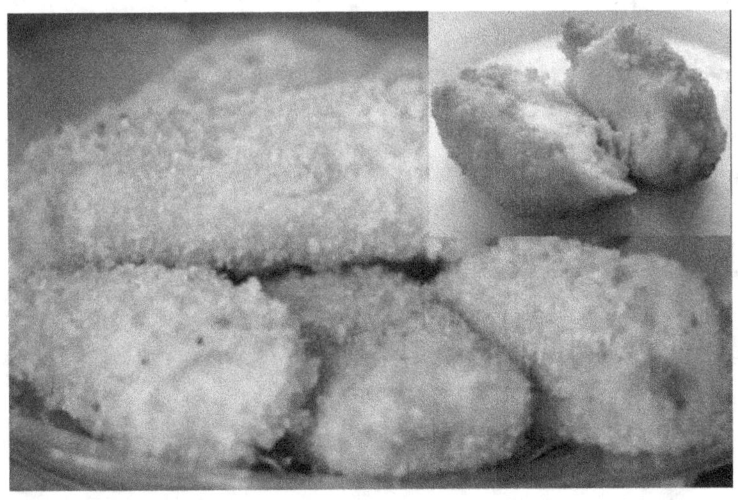

Ingredients

1 pound fresh or frozen crab meat

or A 14.75-ounce can water-packed salmon or tuna.

½ cup unsalted cracker crumbs or plain bread crumb

2 egg whites

¼ cup chopped onion

½ teaspoon black pepper

1 tablespoon olive oil or cooking spray

2 tablespoons lemon juice (optional)

½ teaspoon ground mustard (crab only)

¼ cup regular mayonnaise (crab and tuna only)

Preparations

1. Drain the water from canned meat.

2. Combine all above-listed ingredients except oil in a big bowl. Mix well.

3. Make into eight separate balls, and then flatten to form patties.

4. Place a large skillet and pour some oil in it. Heat it up for some minutes.

5. Place patties in hot oil.

6. Fry until brown and flip the other side too. Drain patties on paper towel.

Nutritional Information

189 calories 0g trans fat 337 mg sodium

14g protein 81 mg cholesterol 184 mg potassium

8g total fat 11g carbohydrate 191 mg phosphorus

2g saturated fat 1gram fiber 124 mg calcium

Baked Fish

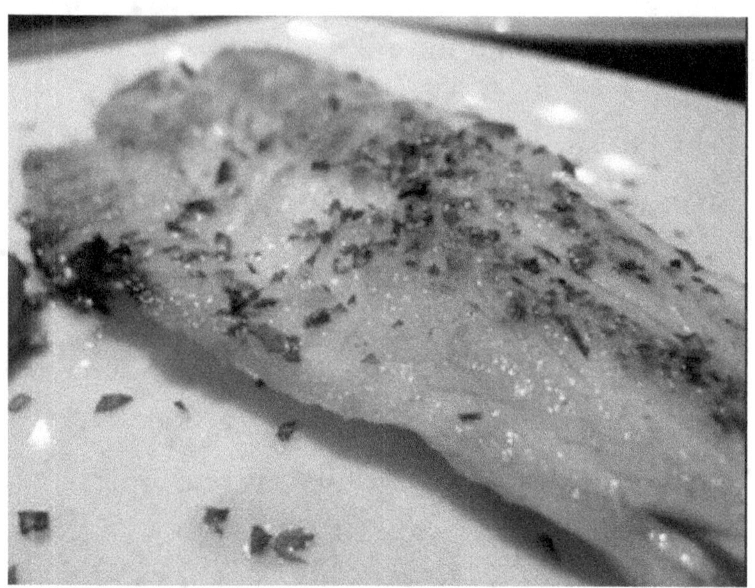

Ingredients

Four 3-ounce trout fillets or any other baking fish

1 ½ teaspoon black pepper

1 tablespoon garlic powder

2 tablespoons parmesan cheese

1 ½ teaspoon paprika

¼ medium green pepper

1 small onion

1 small lemon

Preparations

1. Preheat your oven to 380°F.

2. Gently grease a cooking pan and add your fish.

3. Sprinkle garlic powder, paprika, and black pepper on both sides of the fish.

4. Pour some Squeeze juice of lemon onto fish.

5. Chop some green pepper and onions then spread on the fish.

6. Bake for 30 minutes.

7. When fish is done, sprinkle parmesan cheese and Serve hot.

Nutritional Information

164 calories 0g trans fat 86 mg sodium

20g   protein 62 mg cholesterol 452 mg potassium

6g fat 8g carbohydrate 252 mg phosphorus

1g saturated 3g fiber 80 mg calcium

Yield: 4

Shrimp Salad

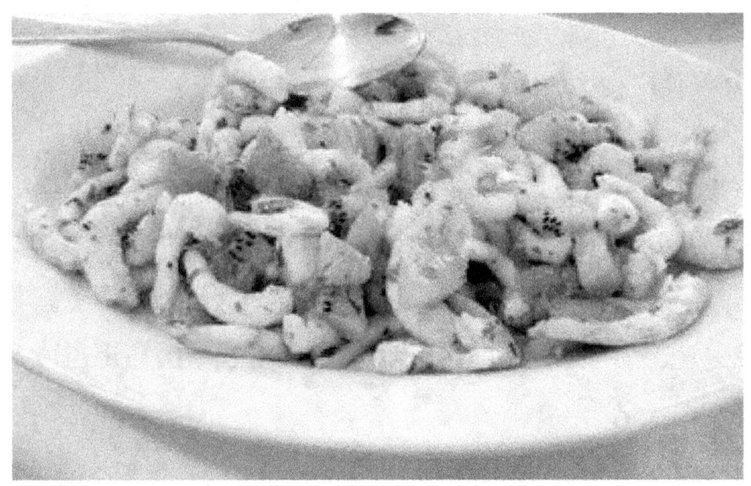

Ingredients

1 pound shrimp, boiled, chopped and deveined

1 hardboiled egg, chopped

1 tablespoon celery, chopped

1 tablespoon green pepper, chopped

1 tablespoon onion, chopped

2 tablespoon mayonnaise

1 teaspoon lemon juice

½ teaspoon chili powder

⅛ teaspoon hot sauce

½ teaspoon dry mustard lettuce, shredded or chopped

Preparations

1. Put all ingredients except lettuce in a bowl to mix; then mix well.

2. Keep it in refrigerator for 30 minutes.

3. Serve as a salad and garnish with lettuce, if desired, or serve on a sandwich.

Nutritional Information

157 calories 0g trans fat 232 mg sodium

26g protein 234 mg cholesterol 233 mg potassium

5g total fat 1gram carbohydrate 263 mg phosphorus

1g saturated fat 0g fiber 67 mg calcium

Yield: 4

Seafood Supreme

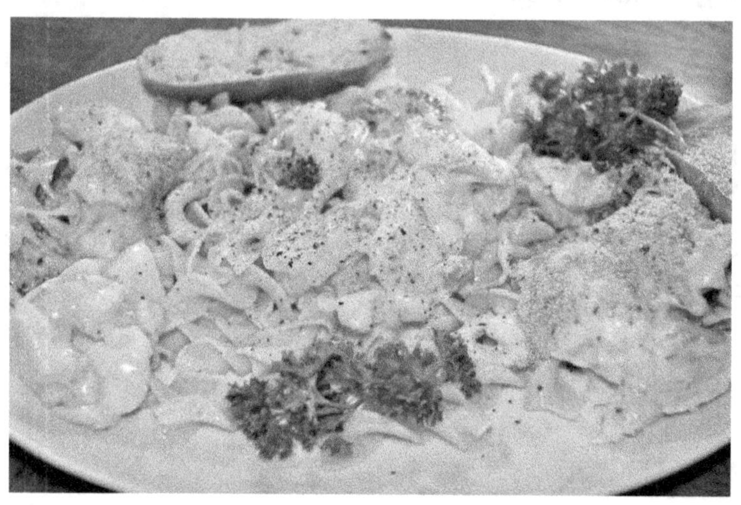

Ingredients

1 cup of crabmeat, cooked (boiled)

1 cup of shrimp, cooked (boiled)

4 tablespoon green pepper, chopped

2 tablespoon green onions, chopped

1 cup of celery, chopped

½ cup frozen green peas

½ teaspoon black pepper

½ cup of mayonnaise

1 cup of bread crumbs

Preparations

1. Preheat oven to 375°F.

2. Put all ingredients except bread crumbs in
   a bowl then mix.

3. Keep in a greased casserole dish.

4. Add your bread crumbs.

5. Bake for 30 minutes.

Nutritional Information

220 calories 0g trans fat 445 mg sodium 16g protein 28 mg cholesterol 255 mg potassium 8g   total fat 20g   carbohydrate 148 mg phosphorus 1gram saturated fat 2g fiber 85 mg calcium

Yield: 6

Crab Cakes

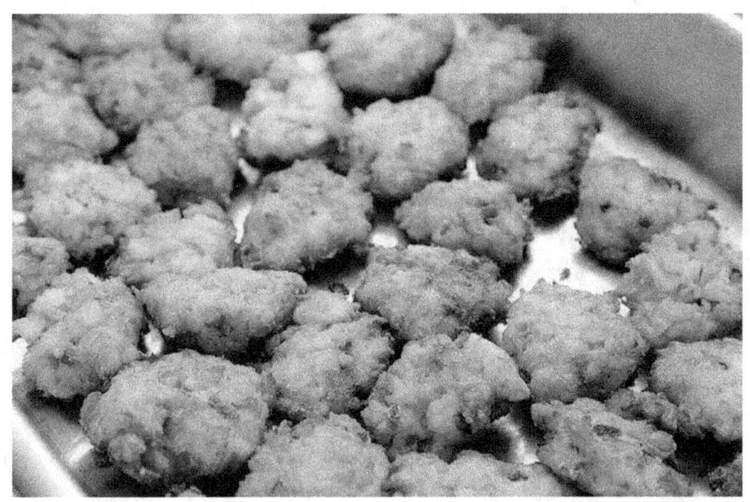

Ingredients

1 egg

⅓ cup of red or green pepper, finely chopped

⅓ cup of low sodium crackers

¼ cup of reduced fat mayonnaise

1 teaspoon garlic powder

1 teaspoon crushed red pepper or black pepper

2 tablespoons lemon juice

1 tablespoon dry mustard

2 tablespoon olive oil

Preparations

1. Combine all your ingredients.

2. Split into six balls and form patties.

3. Pour some olive oil in pan and heat at medium heat or oven at 350°F.

4. Fry balls for 4-5 minutes or bake 15 minutes in the oven.

5. Serve when done

Nutritional Information

101 calories 0g trans fat 67 mg sodium

2g protein 41 mg cholesterol 72 mg potassium

9g total fat 5g carbohydrate 43 mg phosphorus

1g saturated fat 0g fiber 16 mg calcium

Yield: 6

Fish Tacos

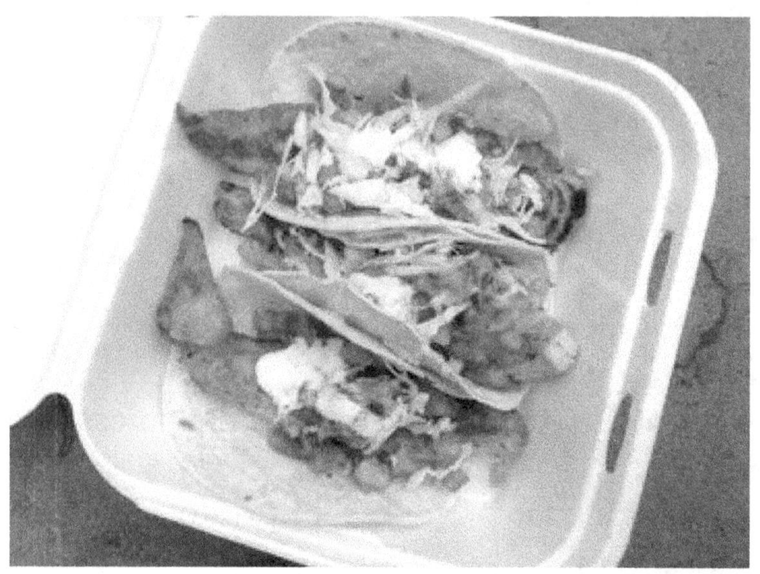

Ingredients

13-15 fish fillets or tilapia or as desired

¼ cup of unsalted butter or margarine

2 teaspoon dill weed

1 teaspoon garlic powder

¼ cup of lemon juice

20 saltine crackers, unsalted tops, crushed finely

Preparations

1. Preheat oven to 400°F.

2. Mix your crackers, garlic, and grill.

3. Toss in some butter and melt butter.

4. Dip your fish in melting butter and crumbs and roll it up, ensuring its well.

5. Place in baking pan and bake 8-10 minutes

Nutritional Information

164 calories 0g trans fat 138 mg sodium

21g   protein 57 mg cholesterol 335 mg potassium

6g   total fat 7g   carbohydrate 181 mg phosphorus

4g saturated fat 0g fiber 23 mg calcium

Yield: 4

Tuna-Noodle

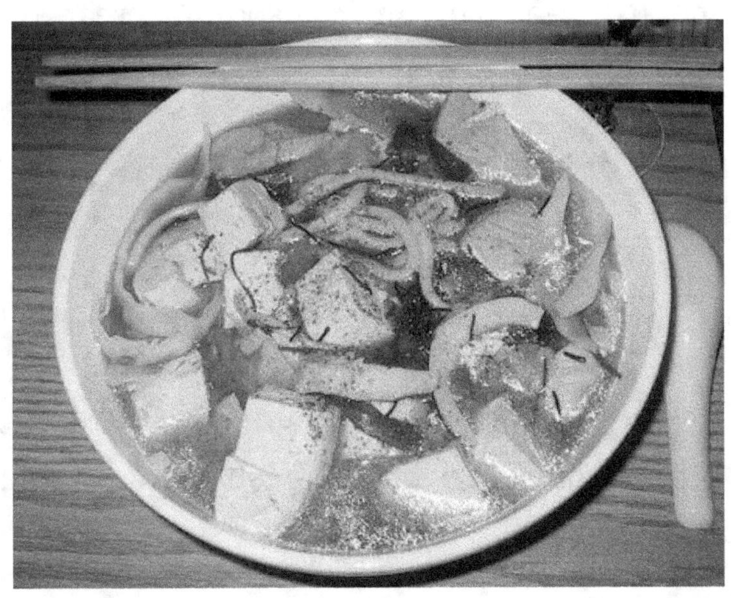

Ingredients

2 tablespoons minced fresh onion

⅔ cup of water

¼ teaspoon curry powder

¼ teaspoon black pepper

Olive cooking spray

One 10 ¾-ounce can low sodium cream of mushroom soup, undiluted

2 cups of hot cooked rotini (corkscrew pasta, cooked without salt or fat)

½ cup frozen green peas, thawed

One 9 ¼-ounce low sodium albacore tuna, with drained, chopped, fresh parsley and water. (optional)

Preparations

1. Get a large skillet and spread some cooking spray over it. Set it on medium heat

2 Chop your onion and toss it in then fry until soft.

3. Mix the water, curry powder, pepper, and soup in a bowl; stir and add to skillet.

4. Pour cooked rotini, peas, and tuna; mix well. Cook uncovered, over low heat 10 minutes, while you stir.

5. Garnish with parsley, if desired.

Nutritional information

269 calories 0gram trans fat 407 mg sodium

18g protein 58 mg cholesterol 515 mg potassium

4g total fat 38g carbohydrate 228 mg phosphorus

0g saturated 1gram fiber 30 mg calcium

Yield: 4

Chicken Recipes for Kidney

Oven Fried Chicken

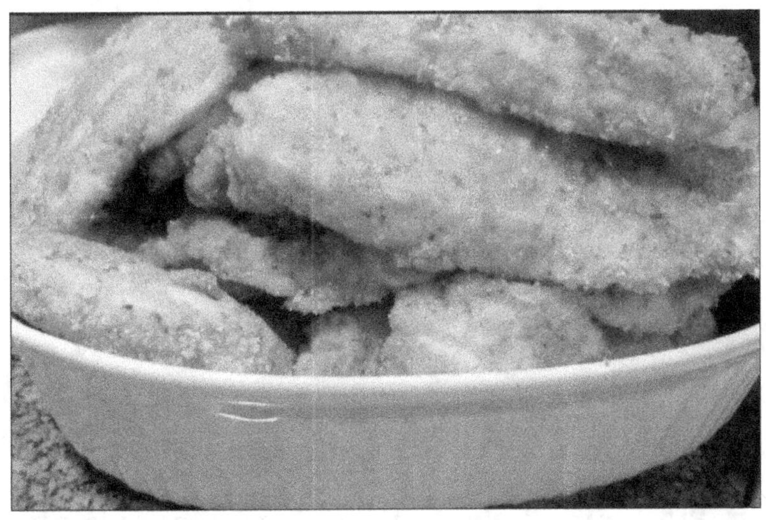

Ingredients

2 ½ pound fryer (cut as desired)

1 tablespoon lemon juice

1 cup all-purpose flour

1 teaspoon black pepper

1 cup corn flakes, crushed

¼ teaspoon poultry seasoning

4 tablespoons olive oil

Preparations

1. Preheat oven to 400°F.

2. Wash chicken very well and dry. Apply some lemon juice on it

3. In a bag, add flour, black pepper, corn flakes, and poultry seasoning. Mix well.

4. Get a cooking or baking pan and grease with olive oil

5. Put your chicken in the bag of ingredients, and shake vigorously

6. Arrange coated chicken in the pan.

7. Cook until Brown then flip the other side and cook in oven 20-30 minutes.

Nutritional Information

280 calories 0g trans fat 74 mg sodium

15g   protein 52 mg cholesterol 150 mg potassium

18g   total fat 15g   carbohydrate 120 mg
phosphorus

3g saturated fat 1gram fiber 12 mg calcium

Yield: 8 (or 8 pieces)

Lemon Chicken

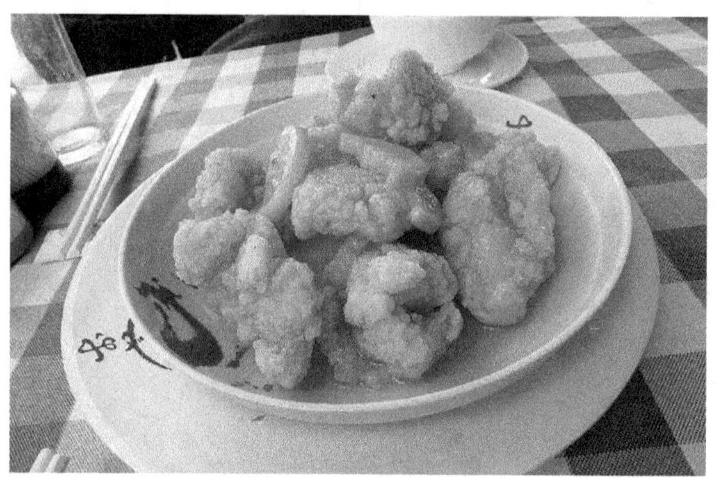

Ingredients

2 ½ pound fryer (cut as desired)

1 tablespoon lemon juice

1 cup all-purpose flour

1 teaspoon black pepper

1 cup corn flakes, crushed

¼ teaspoon poultry seasoning

4 tablespoons olive oil

Preparations

1. Preheat oven to 400°F.

2. Clean and wash your chicken breast thoroughly. Grease it with a lemon juice

3. Get a small bag, combine flour, black pepper, corn flakes, and poultry seasoning?

Shake well.

4. Get a baking pan (about 1" deep), pour some oil

5. Mix in the bag all the ingredient with your chicken

6. Arrange coated chicken in pan.

7. Cook until Brown in oven 20-30 minutes on each side.

Nutritional Information

280 calories 0g trans fat 74 mg sodium

15g protein 52 mg cholesterol 150 mg potassium

18g total fat 15g carbohydrate 120 mg phosphorus

3g saturated fat 1gram fiber 12 mg calcium

Yield: 8 (or 8 pieces)

Chicken and Rice

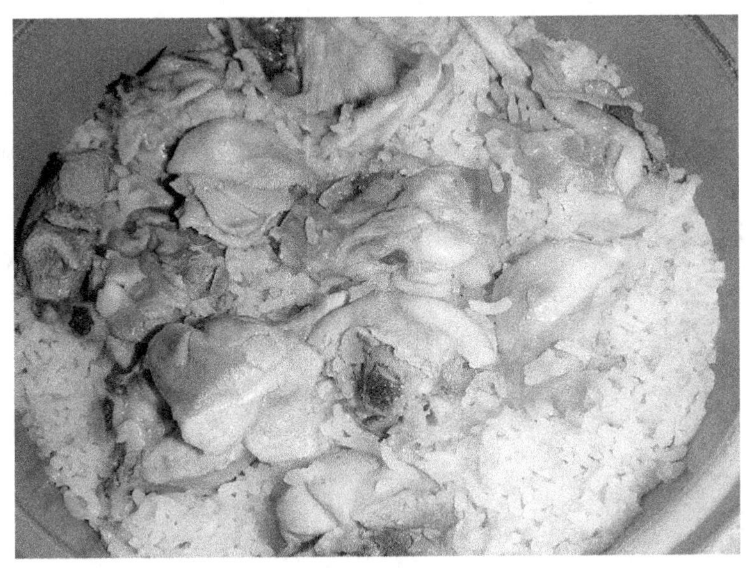

Ingredients

1 pound chicken parts

1 teaspoon black pepper

1 tablespoon poultry seasoning

½ cup of chopped onion

1 teaspoon onion powder

½ teaspoon garlic powder

1 teaspoon crushed bay leaves (optional)

4 cups of water

1 cup of uncooked rice

1 tablespoon olive oil

Preparations

1. Get chicken breast, chop into pieces and mix with the following; black pepper, poultry seasoning, onions, onion powder, and garlic powder, and bay leaves. Transfer them to the Dutch oven; add some water. Cook until chicken is soft and edible.

2. Manually takeaway all the bones from your chicken. When done, keep two cups of chicken broth liquid.

3. Get a large cooking pot and combine rice, olive oil, 2 cups broth, and chicken meat. boil over medium-high heat.

4. Cook on low heat for 20-25 minutes. Serve hot.

Nutritional Information

212 calories 0g trans fat 76 mg sodium

21g protein 60 mg cholesterol 283 mg potassium

8g total fat 11g carbohydrate 218 mg phosphorus

2g saturated 1gram fiber 25 mg calcium

Yield: 6

Chicken Salad Delight

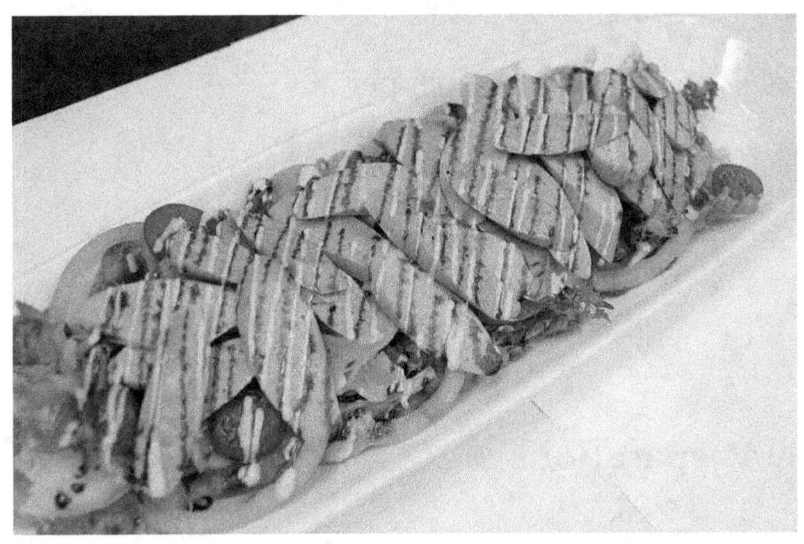

Ingredients

2 cups of chicken, diced

⅓ cup of celery, chopped

¼ cup of fresh onion, chopped

¼ cup of fresh green pepper, chopped

1 teaspoon parsley, dried (optional)

1 tablespoon lemon juice

¼ teaspoon black pepper

1 teaspoon dry mustard

½ cup of mayonnaise

Preparations

1. Combine chicken, parsley, onion, green pepper, celery, and toss with lemon juice. Then set aside

2. Get a bowl and mix black pepper, mustard, and mayonnaise. Add to chicken mixture, Stir to mix.

Nutritional Information

181 calories 1g trans fat 239 mg sodium

18g   protein 47 mg cholesterol 205 mg potassium

10g   total fat 3g   carbohydrate 149 mg phosphorus

2g saturated 0g fiber 16 mg calcium

Yield: 5

Chicken Vegetable Salad

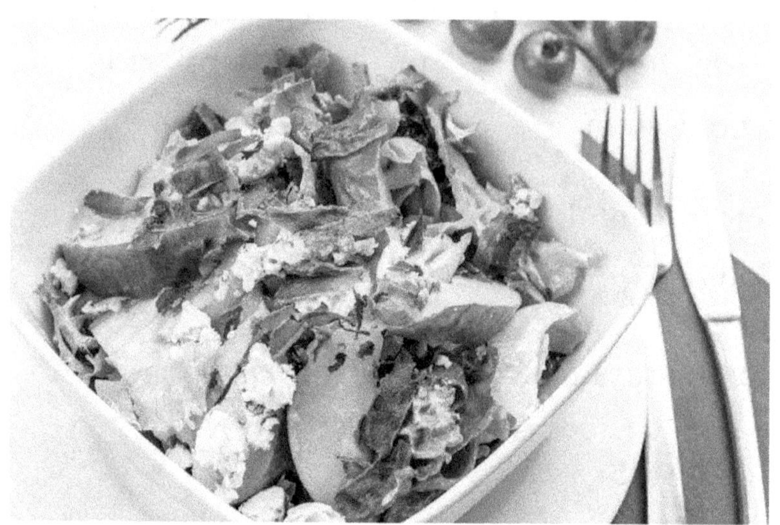

Ingredients

1 ½ cups of cooked chicken, diced

½ cup of green pepper, finely chopped

½ cup of celery, finely diced

½ cup of onions, finely chopped

3 tablespoons pimentos, diced

½ cup of salad dressing or light mayonnaise

1 tablespoon lemon juice

Preparations

1. Get a bowl and mix the following; chicken, green pepper, celery, onions and pimentos.

2. In another bowl, mix mayonnaise and lemon juice. Pour over chicken mixture.

3. Combine well, cover and chill.

4. Serve in a lettuce cups.

Nutritional Information

221 calories 0 trans fat 245 mg sodium

18g   protein 47 mg cholesterol 230 mg potassium

15g fat 15g carbohydrate 143 mg phosphorus

3g saturated fat 0g fiber 22 mg calcium

Yield: 4

Curry Chicken

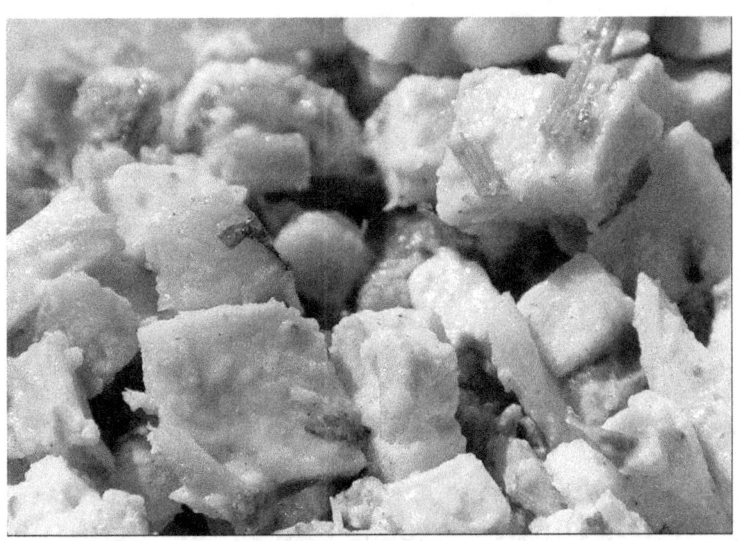

Ingredients

1 skinned chicken cut into small parts.

¼ cup of lemon juice

2 teaspoons curry powder

1 medium onion, chopped

½ teaspoon black pepper

½ teaspoon dry thyme

2 tablespoon vegetable or olive oil

1 cup water

1 medium garlic clove, chopped (optional)

Preparations

1. Get a chicken breast and chop them into smaller bits. Wash, clean, and pat dry. Next, you'll add lemon juice.

2. Combine all seasoning and rub it on chicken.

3. Keep in the refrigerator and allow to marinate for sixty minutes. Or overnight.

4. Heat oil in a saucepan, cook seasoned chicken until there is a color change to brown

5. Rinse the remaining season from the pan with water

6. Pour over browned chicken. Let it cook in low heat until soft.

7. Serve when done with rice

Nutritional Information

323 calories 0g trans fat 93 mg sodium

21g protein 89 mg cholesterol 317 mg potassium

24g total fat 5g carbohydrate 214 mg phosphorus

6g saturated fat 0g fiber 25mg calcium

Yield: 6

Chicken Stew

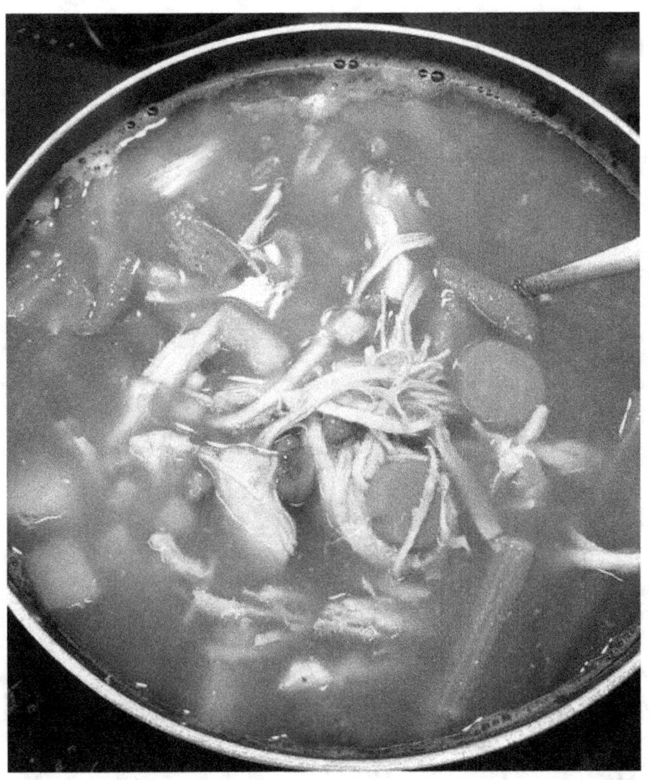

Ingredients

2 pounds chicken breast cut into minute sizes

1 cup sliced onions

¾ cup of green peppers

2 cloves garlic, minced

2 tablespoon all-purpose flour

3 tablespoon olive oil

One 10-ounce bag frozen carrots

¼ teaspoon dried basil

¼ teaspoon black pepper

One 110-ounce bag frozen sliced okra

Two 10 ½-ounce cans low-sodium chicken broth

Preparations

1. Preheat your Dutch oven and add some two tablespoons of oil. Throw in the chicken and over medium high heat.

2. Remove from heat and keep aside. Add remaining one tablespoon of oil

3. Toss in your chopped pepper, garlic, and onion.

4. Add flour and cook 2-3 minutes, stirring constantly.

5. Add chicken and broth, cook until boiling.

6. Add carrots, basil and black pepper, cover and cook in low heat for about 10 minutes. Gravy will become thick end as you cook

7. Add okra and cook for 10-15 minutes.

8. Eat with hot rice

Nutritional Information

142 calories 1gram trans fat 93 mg sodium

10g protein 15 mg cholesterol 453 mg potassium

8g total fat 13g carbohydrates 129 mg phosphorus

1gram saturated fat 3g fiber 69 mg calcium

Yield: 6

Seasoned Pork Chops

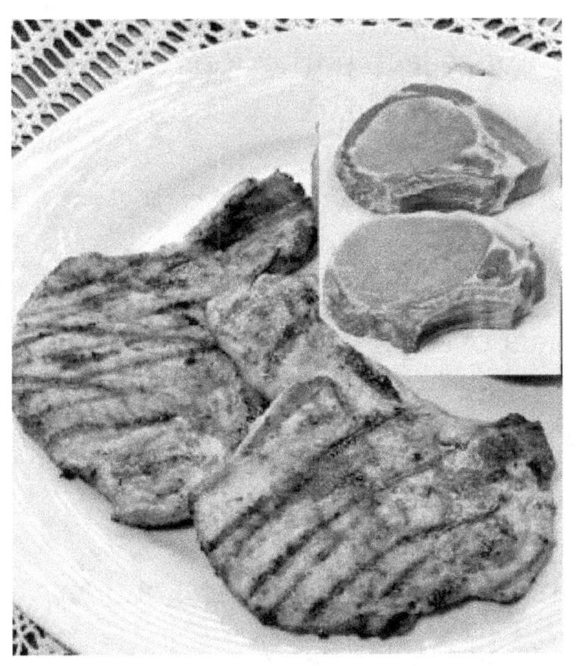

Ingredients

2 tablespoons olive oil

¼ cup of all-purpose flour

1 teaspoon black pepper

½ teaspoon sage

½ teaspoon thyme

Four 4-ounce lean pork chops (fat removed)

Preparations

1. Preheat oven to 350°F.

2. Get a cooking pan and pour two tablespoons of oil in it.

3. Combine your flour, black pepper, thyme, and sage.

4. Throw in the pork chops in flour mixture and arrange in baking pan.

5. Transfer to the oven and cook for about 40 minutes or until soft.

6. Remove from oven. Serve when ready.

Nutritional Information

434 calories 0g trans fat 60 mg sodium

19g protein 79mg cholesterol 332mg potassium

34g total fat 12g carbohydrate 199mg phosphorus

10g saturated fat 0g fiber 35mg calcium

Yield: 4 chops

Homemade Pan Sausage

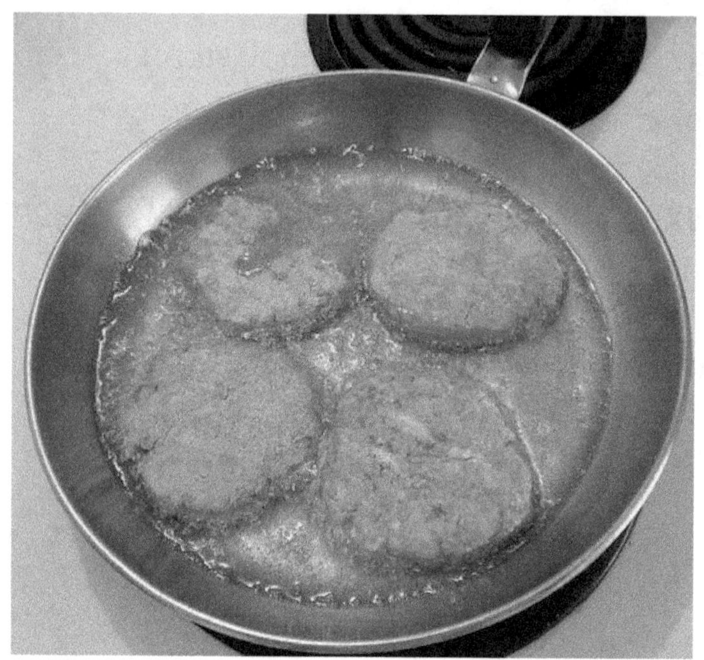

Ingredients

1 pound fresh lean ground pork, beef, chicken or turkey.

2 teaspoons ground sage

2 teaspoons granulated stevia

1 teaspoon ground black pepper

½ teaspoon ground red pepper

1 teaspoon basil (optional) cooking spray

Preparations

1. Let them grind the pork roast or beef loin for you

2. To make sausage, combine all ingredients.

3. Measure two tablespoons of mixed meat and make into a patty.

4. Fry in a kitchen pan until done.

Nutritional Information

96 calories 0g trans fat 22 mg sodium

6g protein 43 mg cholesterol 87 mg potassium

7g total fat 1gram carbohydrate 53 mg phosphorus

2g saturated fat 0g fiber 72 mg calcium

Yield: 12

Spicy Lamb

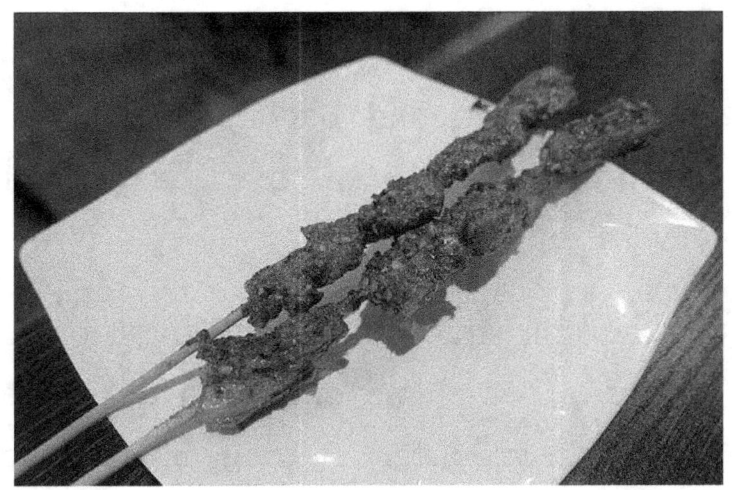

Ingredients

¼ cup of olive oil

1 ½ tablespoon garlic powder

3 teaspoons dry mustard

1 leg of lamb (trimmed for roasting)

Preparations

1. Get a blender and blend ingredients for the marinade: oil, garlic powder and mustard.

2. Get a marinade, and coat lamb legs with it, then refrigerate for six to eight hours or overnight.

3. Arrange a barbeque grill and roast for 30 minutes per pound or until 170°F on a meat thermometer, pouring marinade to coat meat continuously

Nutritional Information

289 calories 0g trans fat 144mg sodium

24g protein 73mg cholesterol 423mg potassium

6g total fat 3g carbohydrate 237mg phosphorus

2g saturated fat 0g fiber 14mg calcium

Yield: 4

Combination Meals

Stuffed green Peppers

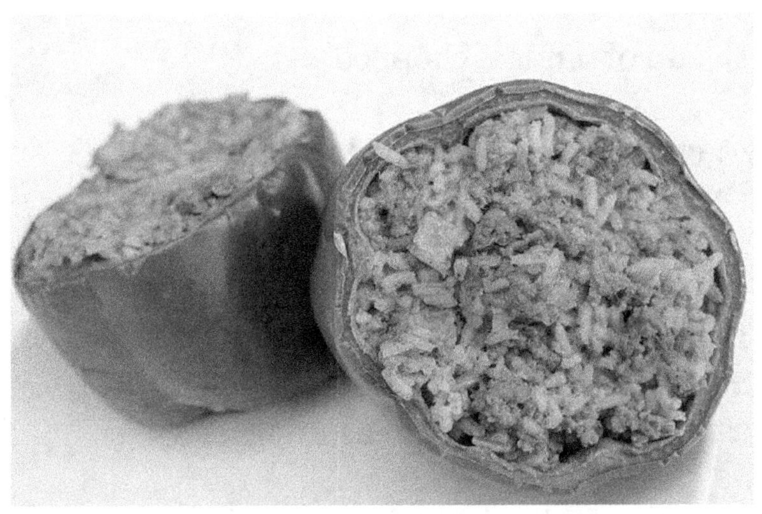

Ingredients

1 ½ cups of cooked rice

6 small green peppers, seeds and tops removed

paprika

2 tablespoon olive oil

½ pound ground chicken, lean beef, or turkey

¼ cup of onions, chopped

¼ cup of celery, chopped

2 tablespoons lemon juice

1 tablespoon celery seed

2 tablespoons Italian seasoning

1 teaspoon black pepper

½ teaspoon stevia

Preparations

1. Preheat oven to 325°F.

2. Set a saucepan, add some olive oil and heat the saucepan.

3. Mix in ground meat, onions and celery, cook until meat is browned.

4. Combine all ingredients except green peppers and paprika to saucepan. Mix well and remove when done

5. Add peppers with mixture. Wrap with aluminum foil or cover while placed in a dish

6. Bake for 30 minutes. Check to see if it's ok and garnish with paprika.

Nutritional Information

131 calories 0g trans fat 36mg sodium

9g protein 28mg cholesterol 160mg potassium

4g total fat 15g carbohydrate 83mg phosphorus

1g saturated fat 1g fiber 38mg calcium

Yield: 6

Rotini with Sausage

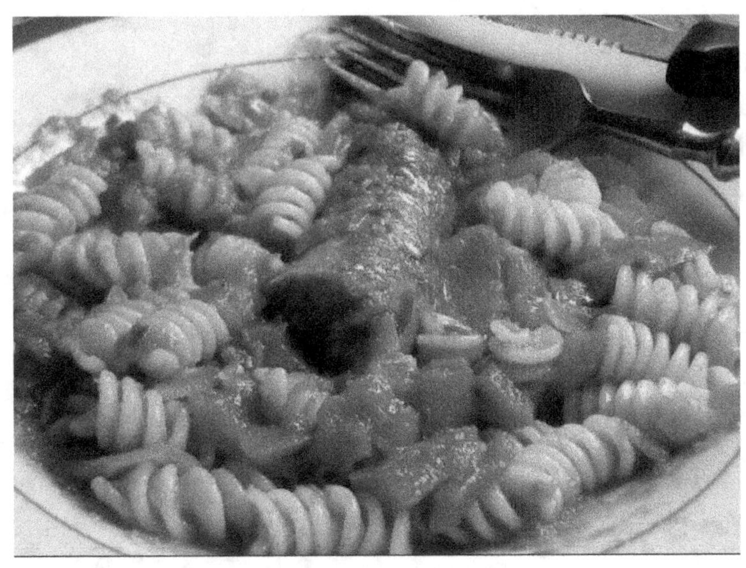

Ingredients

4 ounces uncooked rotini pasta

¾ pound lean ground turkey

1 cup of onion, chopped

1 clove garlic, minced

½ cup of chopped celery

¾ teaspoon Italian seasoning

¼ teaspoon fennel seeds

¼ teaspoon crushed red pepper

2 tablespoons grated parmesan cheese

Preparations

1. Cook rotini pasta according to package Preparations, drain.

2. Cook turkey in a non-stick skillet over medium heat until browned, stirring to crumble.

3. Allow draining on paper towel.

4. Combine to the mix your onion, garlic, celery, and seasonings. And Cook for 3 minutes; stirring occasionally.

5. Serve when done. You may top up with cheese

Nutritional Information

165 calories 0g trans fat 250 mg sodium

13g protein 41mg cholesterol 458mg potassium

2g total fat 28g carbohydrate 161mg phosphorus

1g saturated fat 2g fiber 65 mg calcium

Main dishes

Yield: 4

Eggplant Casserole

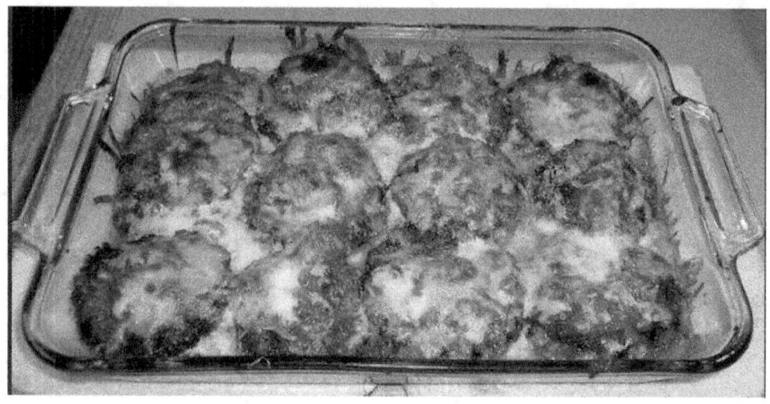

Ingredients

1 large eggplant

2 tablespoon olive oil

½ cup of green pepper, chopped

½ cup of onion, finely chopped

1 pound lean ground beef or turkey

2 cups of plain bread crumbs

1 large egg, slightly beaten

½ teaspoon red pepper, optional

Preparations

1. Preheat oven to 350°F.

2. Broil eggplant until tender; drain and mash.

3. Pour some oil in a cooking pan, heat oil; add green pepper, onion and ground meat. Sauté until cooked.

4. Combine eggplant, bread crumbs, and egg, while mixing well.

5. Pour some red pepper to taste, if desired.

6. Bake a casserole dish for 30-45 minutes.
Serve warm.

Nutritional Information

240 calories 0g trans fat 263 mg sodium

15g protein 74mg cholesterol 380mg potassium

9g total fat 5g carbohydrate 169mg phosphorus

2g saturated fat 4g fiber 71 mg calcium

Yield: 8

Stir Fry Meal

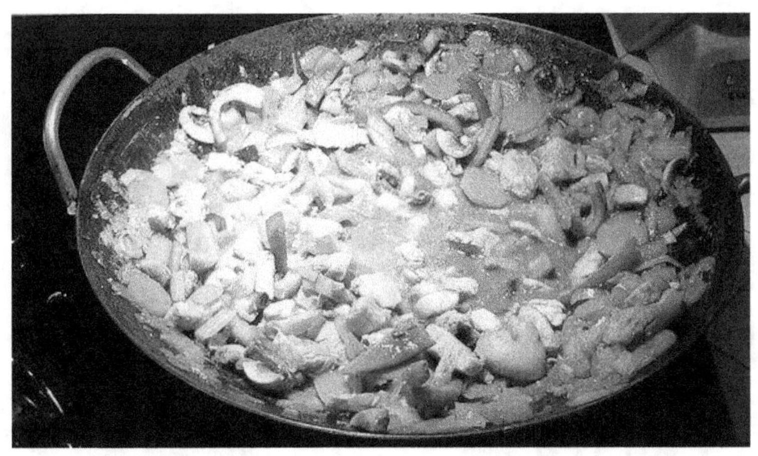

Ingredients

2 tablespoon cooking oil

2 medium chicken breast, cut into bite-size pieces

One 10 ounce package frozen stir fry vegetables

½ tablespoon low sodium soy sauce

2 cups of cooked rice

Preparations

1. Preheat oven and heat up oil in 9-10" skillet
   on high.

2. Add your chicken, and cook.

3. Toss in vegetables.

4. Mix in soy sauce and stir well.

5. Reduce heat to medium-high and cook
   uncovered for 3-5 minutes, or until done,
   stirring frequently.

6. Serve over ⅔ cup rice.

Nutritional Information

315 calories 0g trans fat 37 mg sodium

29g protein 76 mg cholesterol 618 mg potassium

7g total fat 32g carbohydrate 26 mg phosphorus

2g saturated fat 3g fiber 32 mg calcium

Fajitas

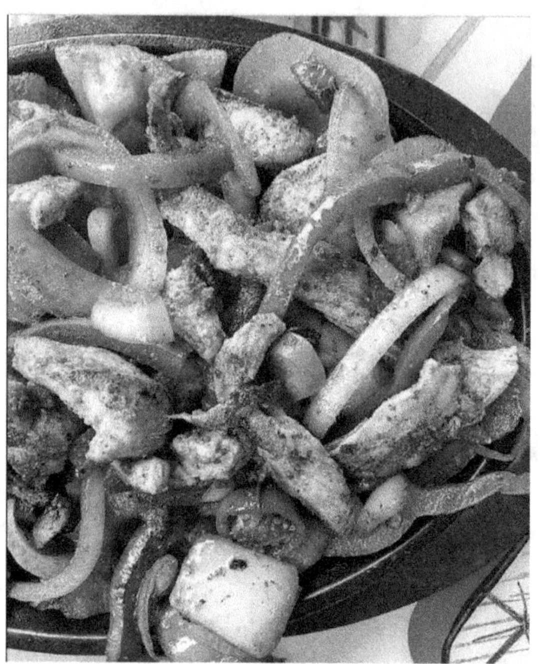

Ingredients

2 tablespoon olive oil

1 ½ pound raw chicken strips or beef strips or shrimp (peeled and deveined)

2 teaspoon chili powder

½ teaspoon cumin

2 tablespoon lemon or lime juice

¼green and/or red pepper sliced lengthwise

½ onion white, sliced lengthwise

½ teaspoon dry cilantro

4 flour tortillas

olive spray

Preparations

1. Preheat oven to 300°F.

2, Pour some oil into a non-stick frying pan over moderate heat.

3. Add your meat, seasonings and lemon/lime juice; cook for 5-10 minutes or until soft.

4. Toss in your pepper and onion into the pan and cook 1-2 minutes.

5. Reduce heat; pour in the cilantro.

6. Place the tortillas on foil and move to oven. Heat for 10 minutes

7. Scoop and share between tortillas, wrap, and serve.

Nutritional Information

184 calories 0g trans fat 121 mg sodium

19g protein 57 mg cholesterol 494 mg potassium

10g total fat 5g carbohydrates 207 mg phosphorus

1gram saturated fat 1gram fiber 38 mg calcium

Yield: 4

Beef and Vegetable Soup

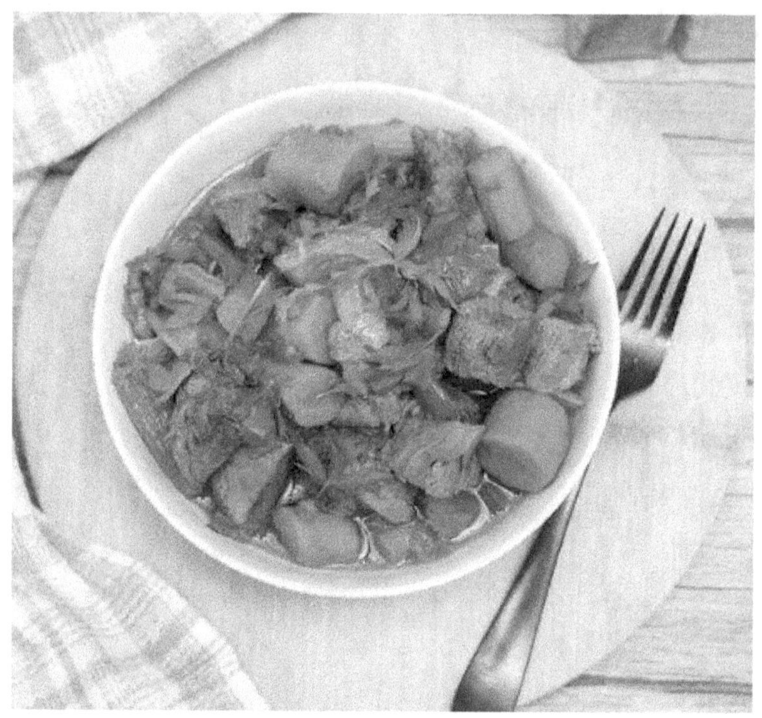

Ingredients

1 pound beef stew

3 ½ cups of water

1 cup of raw sliced onions

½ cup of frozen green peas

1 teaspoon black pepper

½ cup of frozen okra

½ teaspoon basil

½ cup of frozen carrots, diced

½ teaspoon thyme

½ cup of frozen corn

Preparations

1. Place the following; beef stew, onions, black pepper, basil, thyme, and water in a cooking pot. Cook for about 45 minutes.

2. Add your frozen vegetables; cook with low heat until meat is soft. Serve hot.

Nutritional Information

190 calories 0g trans fat 56 mg sodium

11g protein 42mg cholesterol 291mg potassium

13g total fat 7g carbohydrates 121mg phosphorus

5g saturated fat 2g fiber 31mg calcium

Yield: 8

Chicken Noodle Soup

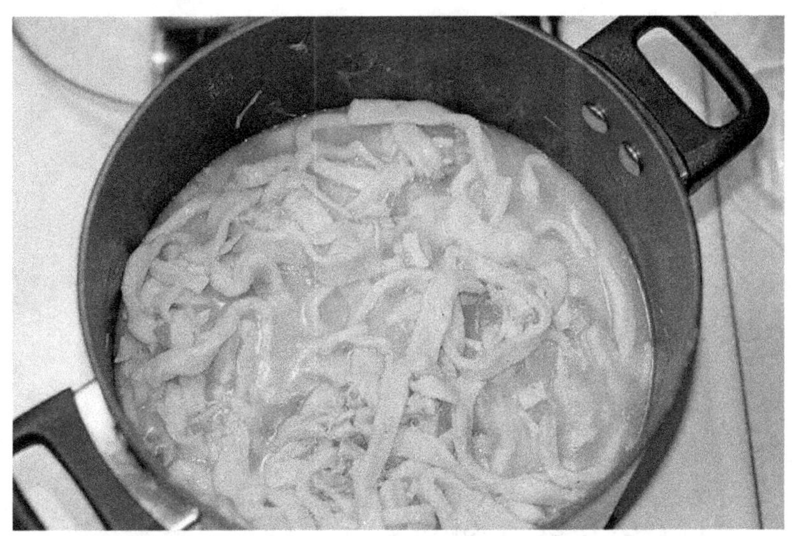

Ingredients

1 pound chicken parts

1 teaspoon red pepper

¼ cup of lemon juice

1 teaspoon caraway seed

3 ½ cups of water

1 teaspoon oregano

1 tablespoon poultry seasoning

1 teaspoon stevia

1 teaspoon garlic powder

½ cup of celery

1 teaspoon onion powder

½ cup of green pepper

2 tablespoons olive oil

1 cup of egg noodles

1 teaspoon black pepper

Preparation

1. Coat chopped chicken with lemon juice.

2. Get a big cooking pot and combine chicken, water, poultry seasoning, garlic powder, onion powder, olive oil, black pepper, red pepper, caraway seed, oregano, and stevia together. Cook for thirty minutes or until chicken meat is soft.

3. Pour in the remaining ingredients and simmer for an additional 15 minutes. Serve hot.

4. You can add more water if desired

Nutritional Information

110 calories 0g trans fat 17 mg sodium

3g protein 12mg cholesterol 101mg potassium

8g fat 7g carbohydrate 39mg phosphorus

2g saturated 0g fiber 21mg calcium

Yield: 8

Herbed Omelet

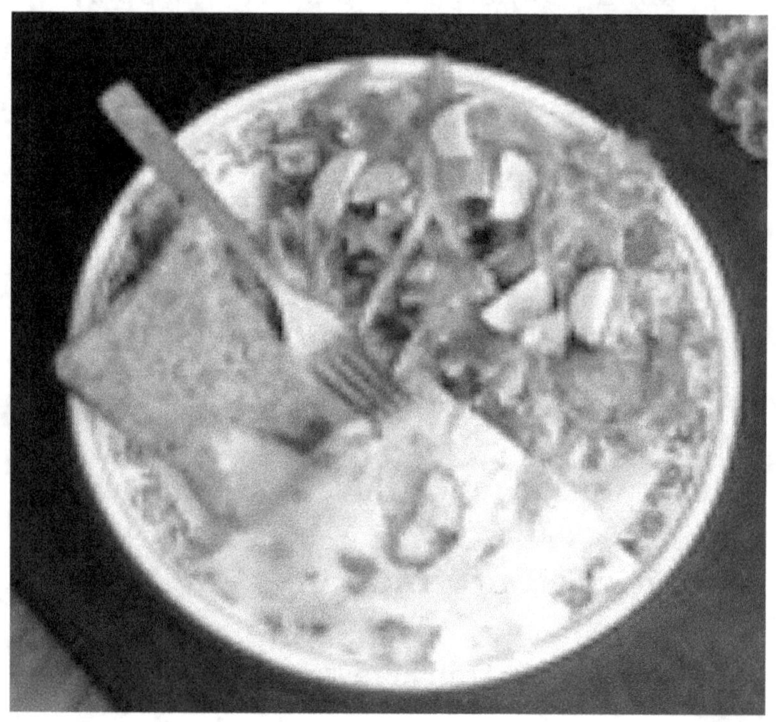

Ingredients

1 ½ teaspoons olive oil

1 tablespoon chopped onion

4 eggs

2 tablespoons water

¼ teaspoon basil

⅛ teaspoon tarragon

¼ teaspoon parsley (optional)

Preparation

1. Begin by beating your eggs. Add some water and spices.

2. Transfer to a cooking pan. Add some oil first, so we heat up in the oil

3. Fry over medium heat

4. As the omelet sets, lift it with a spatula and all the other portion to set

5. Add the cooked onions to the set omelet and transfer from pan to a serving bowl.

Nutritional Information

195 calories 0g trans fat 157 mg sodium

14g protein 474mg cholesterol 157mg potassium

15gram total fat 0g carbohydrate 214mg phosphorus

4g saturated fat 0g fiber 60mg calcium

Side Dishes

Baking Powder Biscuits

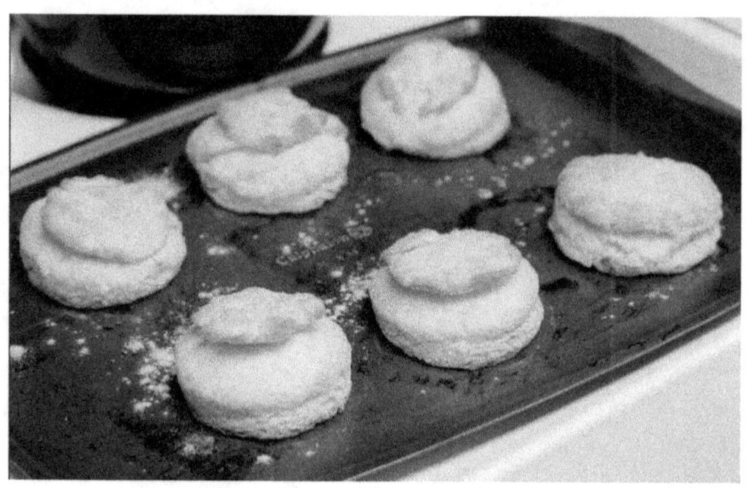

Ingredients

2 cups of all-purpose flour, sifted

3 teaspoons double acting baking powder

2 teaspoons stevia

⅓ cup of vegetable shortening

¼ cup of 1% milk

½ cup of water

Preparation

1. Preheat oven at 350°F.

1. Pour all dry ingredients into a bowl.

2. Make them smaller until crumbs are made. Create a little hole in the middle and pour some milk and water. Stir with a fork until evenly combined

5. The dough should be soft. Transfer unto a smooth flat surface.

6. Knead dough about 10-12 times. You may roll at this point

7. Dip a 2 ½" biscuit cutter into flour; then cut out 10 biscuits.

8. Set a baking sheet and place all the biscuits on it. Bake for 12-15 minutes.

Nutritional Information

162 calories 1g trans fat 150 mg sodium

3g protein 1 mg cholesterol 36 mg potassium

8g total fat 21g carbohydrate 63mg phosphorus

2g saturated fat 1g fiber 92 mg calcium

Yield: 10 biscuits

White Bread Dressing

Ingredients

2 tablespoons margarine

¼ cup of chopped onions

1 ½ cups plain bread crumbs or three slices of bread, crumbled

¼ cup of chopped celery

1 teaspoon poultry seasoning

¼ teaspoon garlic powder

¼ cup of unsalted chicken broth

Preparation

1. Get a small skillet. Add some margarine and heat for three minutes until melts. Add onions. Stir until onions cooked soft.

2. Pour in your bread crumbs, stir it repeatedly to prevent scorching.

3. Remove from heat. Add the following; celery, poultry seasoning garlic powder and chicken broth.

4. Blend well. Place in a small baking pan.

5. Bake for 30 minutes at 375°F.

6. Does it seem dry? Add water to moisten

Nutritional Information

107 calories 0g trans fat 129mg sodium

2g protein 11g carbohydrates 77mg potassium

6g total fat 11mg cholesterol 30mg phosphorus

0g saturated 1g fiber 35mg calcium

Yield: 4

Corn Pudding

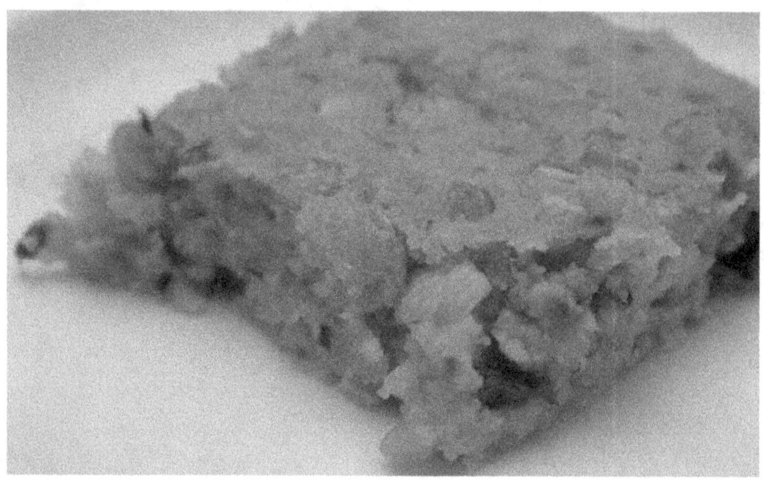

Ingredients

2 cups of kernel corn, canned or fresh cut

3 slightly beaten eggs or ¾ cup egg substitute

½ cup of 1% milk

½ cup of water

⅓ cup of onion, finely chopped

1 tablespoon butter, melted

1 teaspoon granulated stevia

1 teaspoon white or black pepper

Preparations

1. Preheat oven to 350°F.

2. Mix all your ingredients.

3. Transfer into a greased 1 ½-quart casserole dish.

4. Take it to a pan filled with 1 inch of hot water.

5. Bake for about 40-45 minutes,

6. Remove and allow to cool. Serve when done

Nutritional Information

120 calories 0g trans fat 61 mg sodium

6g protein 121mg cholesterol 234mg potassium

5g total fat 17g carbohydrate 122mg phosphorus

2g saturated 2g fiber 49mg calcium

Yield: 6

Rice Casserole

Ingredients

1 cup of white rice, uncooked

2 cups of chicken stock, unsalted

¼ cup of green bell pepper, chopped

½ teaspoon parsley flakes

1 tablespoon olive oil

3 Fresh green onions, chopped

1 tablespoon chives

Preparations

1. Preheat oven to 350°F.

2. Mix all ingredients, and place in a casserole dish.

3. Cover with lid and cook for 45-50 minutes or till liquid is absorbed

4. Remove from heat, allow to cool for ten minutes and serve

Nutritional Information

53 calories 0g trans fat 19 mg sodium

2g protein 7g carbohydrate 74mg potassium

2g total fat 0mg cholesterol 29mg phosphorus

0 saturated 0g fiber 7mg calcium

Tuna Mayonnaise Pasta Salad

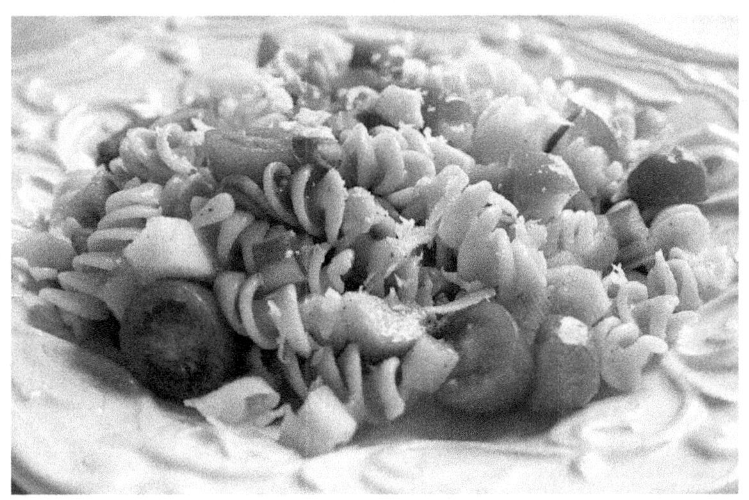

Ingredients

90g/3oz pasta shells

1 x 200g/8oz can of tuna in spring-water

2 spring onions, chopped

2 tablespoons reduced-fat Mayonnaise

2 tablespoons canned sweetcorn in water

Handful parsley or coriander, chopped

Black or white pepper

Preparations

1. Cook the pasta following the instructions on the packet. Drain and put into a large bowl.

2. Drain the tuna and combine with the pasta and the spring onions, parsley and sweetcorn.

3. Pour some mayonnaise and stir until everything is coated.

4. Season with pepper. Garnish with some extra parsley and serve.

Salmon Salad

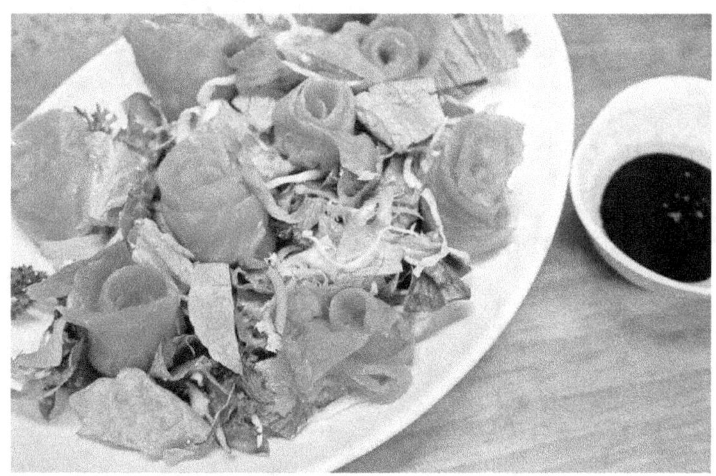

Ingredients

Small tin of salmon, bones removed

4 lettuce leaves, e.g. little gem or

round lettuce

1 spring onion

1/4 bag /1 handful of watercress

2 slices of beetroot

3 rings of red pepper

1 Cauliflower

1 tablespoon of coleslaw

Preparations

1. Slice your Cauliflower into bits. Cleanse with water and transfer into a cooking pot. Set your oven and steam until its tender. Drain.

2. Chop all salad ingredients into small chunks and mix very well.

3. Transfer the salad and Cauliflower on a plate.

4. Arrange the coleslaw and salmon in the middle of the plate and serve.

Serves 1

Meat Pasties

Ingredients

1 packet (500g/1lb) shortcrust pastry

200g/8oz minced beef (low fat if possible)

1 small (100g) Cauliflower

1 medium carrot

1 small onion

White or black pepper

Dried herbs (optional)

Preparation

1. Preheat the oven to 200°C/400°F/. Get a cooking pan. Add your meat and cook until brown

2. Pour in some water to half cover the meat and cook on low heat for 15 minutes. Drain to take away excess liquid.

3. Now it's time to boil Cauliflower. Pour your Cauliflower into a cooking pot. Add your onion and boil for ten minutes. Remove from heat. Drain off water and mash.

4. Pour into the mince. Check the taste of the meat. Season with pepper and other seasonings as desired. Split and share the meat between the rounds of Pastry.

5. Dampen edges and press to fold the edges. Transfer to a baking tray after dipping in milk. Bake for 25-30 minutes in the oven.

6. Serve when done

Serves 6

Chicken Tikka

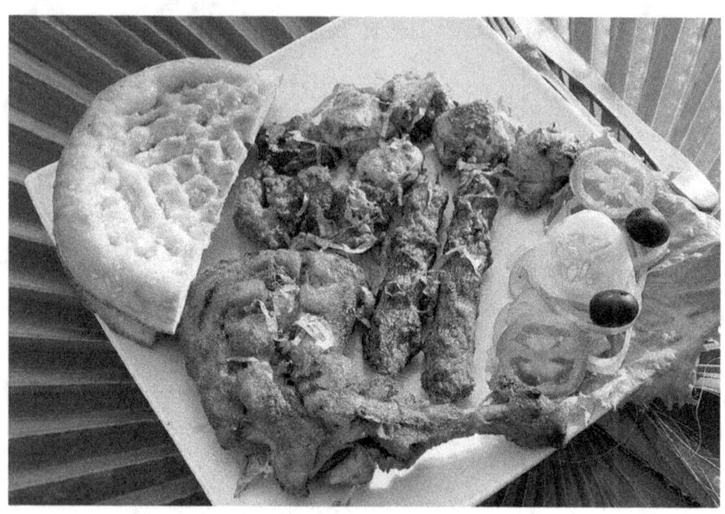

Ingredients

3 tablespoons of low-fat natural yogurt

1 tablespoon curry paste

1 teaspoon lemon juice

2 small boneless chicken breasts, skin removed

Preparation

1. Pour your curry paste into the yogurt.

2. Get a bowl, transfer your chicken into a bowl and add the lemon juice and curried yogurt.

3. Allow to sit for one hour, or overnight in the fridge; So all your flavors infuse. That's why we are leaving it this long.

4. Transfer the coated chicken to a grill and heat your grill place the chicken and grill for twenty minutes.

5. Check and piece with a knife

6. Serve and garnish with tortilla wraps or other toppings

Serves 2 (as a main meal)

Serves 4 (as a snack)

Chicken with Apple and Ginger

Ingredients

4 skinless chicken breasts or legs

1 tablespoon mustard

1 tablespoon honey

3 tablespoons apple juice

Grate 1 apple

2 teaspoons ground ginger powder

Preparation

1. Preheat oven to 190°C/375°F/Gas Mark 5.

2. Chop and slice in threes your chicken.

3. Combine your mustard, honey, apple juice, apple zest and ground ginger and pour over the chicken using a spoon

4. Cook in the pre-heated oven for 25-30 minutes, or until thoroughly cooked.

5. Serve when done with rice or bread and vegetables you prefer.

Serves 4

Steak with Peppercorn Sauce

Ingredients

2 x 125g/4oz beef steaks

100g/4oz half-fat crème Fraiche or double cream

2 teaspoons olive oil

Freshly ground black pepper

2 teaspoons peppercorns, crushed

Preparation

1. Set a cooking pan and add some oil, allow to heat up then add steaks. Sprinkle some black pepper to taste bring down the

steaks from the pan, allow to cool for some time.

2. Add the peppercorns to the frying pan and stir continuously simmer gently for 2 minutes until the sauce thickens.

3. Scoop out 1-2 tablespoons of sauce over each of the steak.

4. Serve immediately with salad or boiled vegetables of your choice.

Serves 2

Pork Chops with Herb Crust

Ingredients

2 pork chops (fat trimmed off)

1 teaspoon mustard

2 teaspoon oil

2 spring onions or 1 shallot, finely chopped

1 clove garlic, crushed

2 tablespoons of fresh or bought breadcrumbs

1 pinch mixed dried herbs or a handful of fresh herbs (e.g. parsley) chopped.

Preparation

1. Preheat the oven to 200°C/400°F/

2. Get a baking dish and spread your mustard over each side of the pork.

3. For herb crust, combine your oil, onions, garlic, dried herbs, and breadcrumbs.

4. Hand Press the herb crust mixture on each pork chop/loin and cover the dish with tin foil.

5. Bake for 25 minutes, take out the foil for the last 5 minutes.

6. Serve when done with any vegetable.

Serves 2

Blueberry Baked Bread

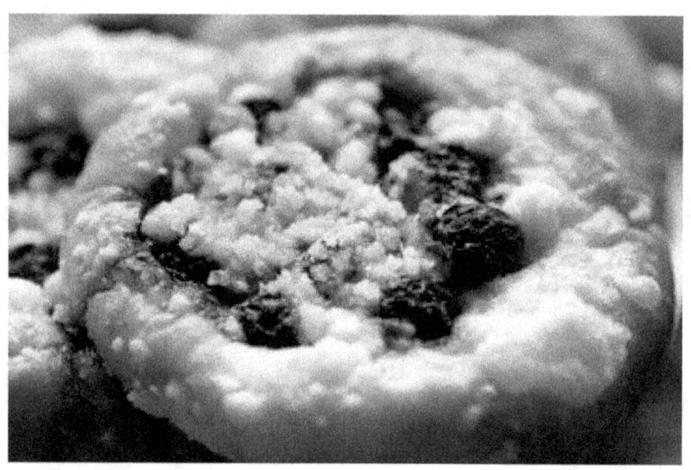

Ingredients

1 quart blueberries, fresh or frozen

¼ cup of water (omit if berries are frozen)

1 teaspoon lemon juice

½ cup of stevia

1 pinch nutmeg

1 pinch cinnamon

1 tablespoon margarine

3 slices bread, buttered and sprinkled with cinnamon and stevia on both sides

Preparation

1. Heat oven to 425°F.

2. Wash blueberries under cool running water.

3. Combine all ingredients in a saucepan except bread. Bring to a boil.

4. Pour blueberry mixture into a shallow baking pan; top with bread cut in halves.

5. Bake until brown (about 10 minutes).

Nutritional Information

176 calories 0g trans fat 92 mg sodium

2g protein 0 mg cholesterol 83 mg potassium

3g total fat 39g carbohydrate 20 mg phosphorus

0g saturated fat 3g fiber 56 mg calcium

Yield: 6

Steamed Asparagus

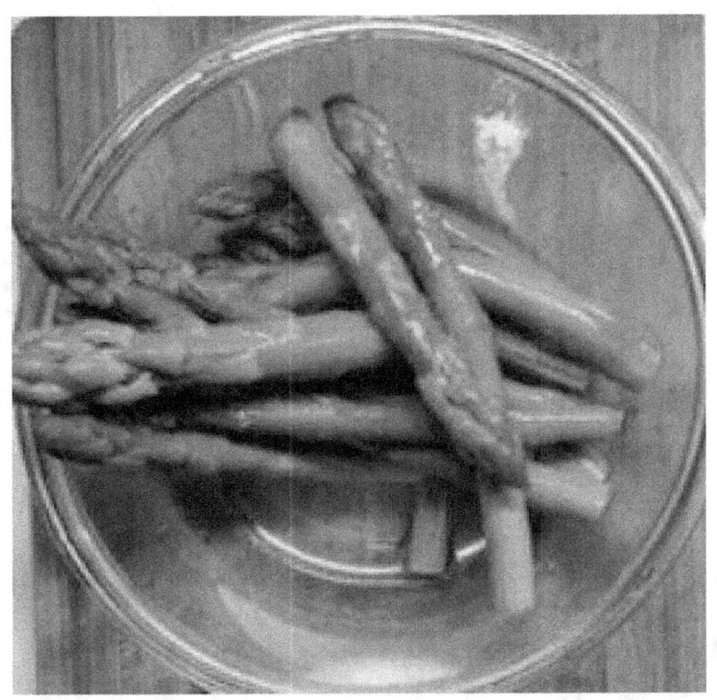

Ingredients

1 tablespoon lemon juice

2 tablespoons margarine, melted (unsalted)

2 cups of water

12 fresh asparagus spears

Preparations

1. Combine lemon juice with margarine; keep aside.

2. Pour some water in a steamer and boil.

3. Add asparagus in a steamer over boiling water.

4. Place in steam for 2 minutes. Do not allow to cook.

5. Remove it from heat and pour margarine with lemon juice over asparagus.

Nutritional Information

62 calories 0g trans fat 1 mg sodium

1g protein 0 mg cholesterol 123 mg potassium

6g total fat 3g carbohydrate 32 mg phosphorus

1g saturated fat 1gram fiber 16mg calcium

Yield: 4

Coleslaw

Ingredients

1 cup cabbage, shredded

2 tablespoons green pepper, chopped

¼ cup of onion, chopped

¼ cup of carrots, shredded

¼ cup of mayonnaise

2 tablespoons vinegar

1 tablespoon stevia

½ teaspoon black pepper

½ teaspoon celery seed (optional)

⅛ teaspoon dill weeds (optional)

Preparations

1. Mix all vegetables.

2. Blend your mayonnaise, vinegar, and seasonings.

3. Add them to the vegetables and toss to mix very well.

Nutritional Information

127 calories 0g trans fat 81 mg sodium

0g protein 0 mg cholesterol 76 mg potassium

11g total fat 6g carbohydrate 14 mg phosphorus

2g saturated fat 1gram fiber 13 mg calcium

Yield: 4

Vegetables & Rice

Ingredients

2 ½ cups of rice, cooked, salt-free

1 10-ounce package frozen green peas, cooked and drained

1 medium onion, chopped

¼ cup of margarine, unsalted

1 tablespoon lemon juice

½ teaspoon thyme

2 tablespoons liquid smoke (optional)

Preparations

1. Preheat your oven and place a cooking pan on it. Slice in some onion and cook onion in margarine until soft.

2. Combine rice, green peas, lemon juice, thyme, and liquid smoke.

3. Cook for 5 minutes.

Nutritional Information

194 calories 0g trans fat 32 mg sodium

4g protein 0mg cholesterol 99 mg potassium

8g total fat 26g carbohydrate 67mg phosphorus

2g saturated fat 3g fiber 23mg calcium

Yield: 6

Macaroni Salad

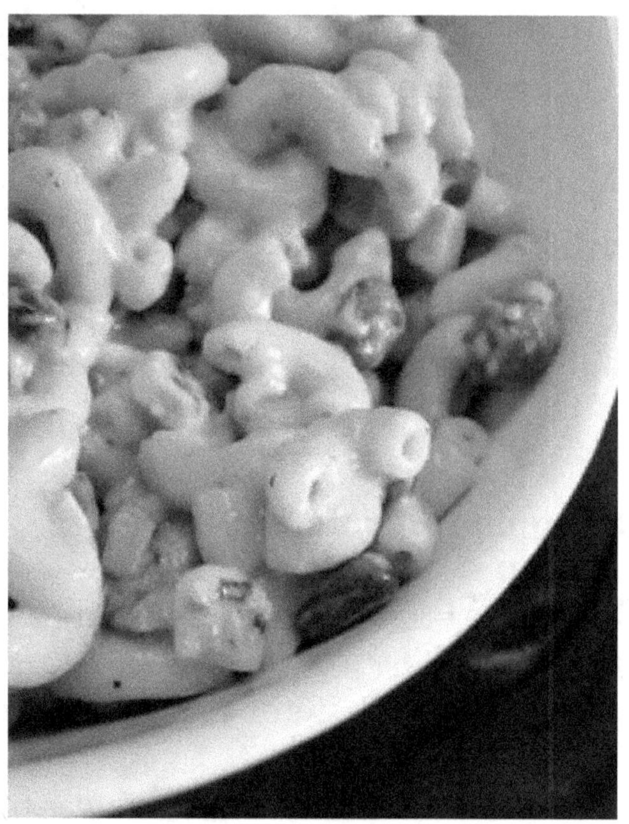

Ingredients

3 cups of macaroni, cooked

¼ cup of pimentos

½ cup of onion, chopped

½ cup of green pepper, chopped

3 hard-boiled, shelled eggs, chopped

½ cup of mayonnaise

½ cup of celery, chopped

1 teaspoon dry mustard paprika

Black pepper

Preparations

1. Rinse cooked macaroni under cold water; drain well.

2. Mix macaroni with other ingredients except for paprika and black pepper. Toss very well.

3. Now Sprinkle with paprika and black pepper.

4. Serve when done

Nutritional Information

223 calories 0g trans fats 103mg sodium

6g protein 80mg cholesterol 106mg potassium

14g total fat 18g carbohydrate 74mg phosphorus

2g saturated fat 2g fiber 20 mg calcium

Green Beans

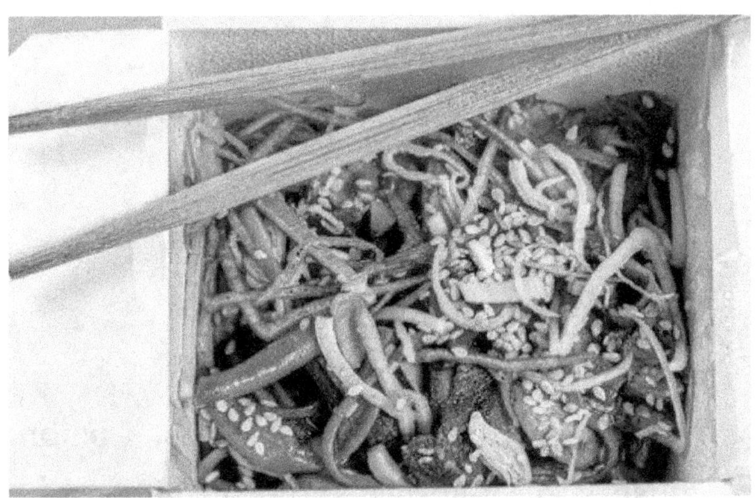

Ingredients

2 cans of whole green beans, drained and rinsed

1 small onion, chopped

½ cup of fresh mushrooms, sliced

1 teaspoon paprika

¼ teaspoon coarse black pepper

1 ½ cups of unsalted top cracker crumbs

4 tablespoons margarine, unsalted

Preparations

1. Preheat oven to 350°F.

2. Mix together green beans, onion, mushrooms, paprika, and black pepper.

3. Get a baking dish and pour the mixture.

4. Top up the mixture with cracker crumbs and margarine.

5. Place in the oven and bake for about 30-35 minutes.

Nutritional Information

137 calories 0g trans fat 77 mg sodium

2g protein 0mg cholesterol 214mg potassium

9g total fat 14g carbohydrate 38mg phosphorus

2g saturated fat 2g fiber 38 mg calcium

Yield: 6

Fried Onion Rings

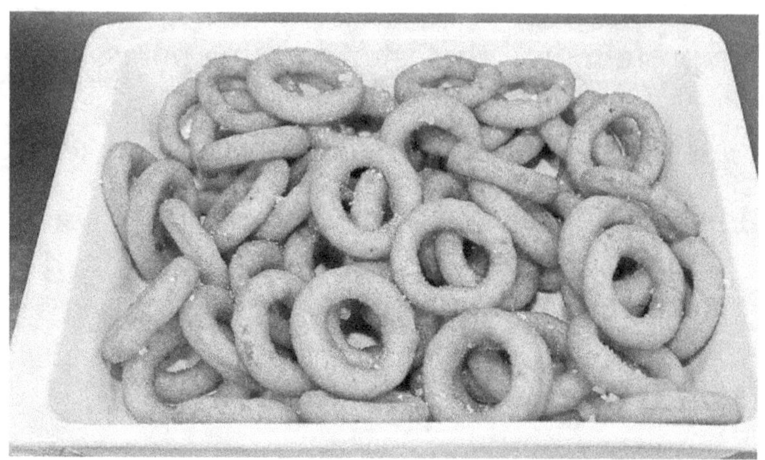

Ingredients

¾ cup of plain cornmeal

¼ cup of all-purpose flour

1 teaspoon stevia

4 medium onions

1 egg, beaten

¼ cup of water

½ cup of olive oil for frying

Preparations

1. Combine your cornmeal, flour and stevia; and keep aside.

2. Peel onions, and slice in rings shape.

3. Combine eggs already beaten egg and water.

4. Dip onion rings in egg wash, then into cornmeal mixture.

5. Fry for 3-5 minutes in heated olive oil, stir until brown.

6. Transfer on a paper towel and allow to drain off. Serve warm when ready.

Nutritional Information

162 calories 0g trans fat 11 mg sodium

2g protein 14g carbohydrate 99 mg potassium

11g total fat 27 mg cholesterol 39 mg phosphorus

1gram saturated fat 2g fiber 11 mg calcium

Yield: 10

Baked Yellow Squash

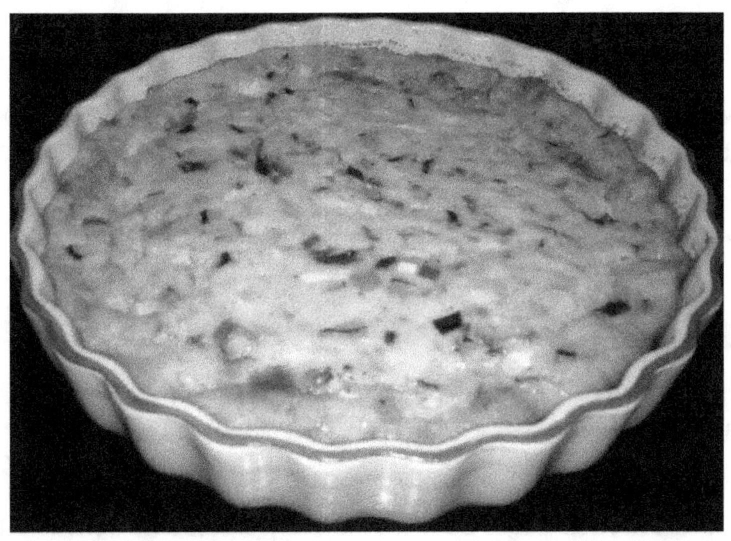

Ingredients

2 tablespoons margarine or butter, melted

¾ teaspoon thyme

⅛ teaspoon black pepper

2 cans yellow squash, sliced

1 medium onion, chopped

1 small stalk celery, chopped

1 large bell pepper, chopped

1 tablespoon lemon juice

Preparations

1. Preheat oven to 350°F.

2. Cook all ingredients except lemon juice in margarine. Cook until onions are translucent.

3. Pour in your lemon juice.

4. Place cooked mixture in a casserole dish.

5. Bake for about 30 minutes. Serve warm when done.

Nutritional Information

49 calories 1g trans fat 34 mg sodium

1g protein 0 mg cholesterol 139 mg potassium

3g total fat 5g carbohydrate 25 mg phosphorus

1g saturated fat 2g fiber 31 mg calcium

Yield: 6

Yellow Squash and Green Onions

Ingredients

2 cups of yellow straight neck or crook neck squash, washed and sliced

2 tablespoons butter or margarine

1 cup of green onion, chopped

1 teaspoon black pepper

Preparations

1. Cook your sliced squash in boiling water for 15 minutes or until soft; drain.

2. Set a saucepan in the oven and heat up. Add some butter and melt throw in some onions and stir until tender.

3. Toss in your squash and black pepper.

4. Cover with a lid cook on low heat for about 5 minutes. Serve when done.

Nutritional Information

87 calories 1gram trans-fat 347 mg sodium

1.5gram protein 0 mg cholesterol 204 mg potassium

8g total fat 4g carbohydrate 40 mg phosphorus

2g saturated fat 2g fiber 31mg calcium

Yield: 3

Green Garden Salad

Ingredients

4 cups of red leaf or other lettuce, shredded

1 carrot, sliced

2 celery stalks, sliced

2 cucumbers, sliced

2 radishes, sliced

1 large bell pepper, diced or sliced into rings

Preparations

1. Combine all vegetables in a large bowl and
   toss.

2. Serve with your favorite salad dressing.

Nutritional Information

30 calories 0g trans fat 20 mg sodium

1gram protein 0 mg cholesterol 215 mg potassium

0g total fat 4g carbohydrate 29 mg phosphorus

0 saturated fat 1gram fiber 25 mg calcium

Yield: 6 cups

Marinated Vegetables

Preparations

1. Using a small size saucepan, combine marinade ingredients, and cook until it is boiled. Allow complete cooling.

2. Mix salad ingredients together.

3. Pour cooled marinade over vegetables and stir.

4. Place in a covered container and refrigerate overnight before serving.

Nutritional Information

85 calories 0g trans fat 13 mg sodium

1g protein 154 mg potassium 0 mg cholesterol

0g total fat 39 mg phosphorus 20g carbohydrate

0g saturated fat 2g fiber 12 mg calcium

Yield: 15

Salt-Free Sweet Brown Mustard

Ingredients

2 teaspoons cornstarch

1 cup of cider vinegar

½ cup of dry mustard

½ cup of stevia powder

½ teaspoon white pepper (or black pepper)

Preparations

1. Pour cornstarch into a bowl containing some vinegar.

2. Preheat your oven. Place a cooking saucepan in it and add the following

ingredients - mustard, stevia, and pepper. Keep stirring until it dissolves.

3. Next pour your cornstarch and cook until thickened. Reduce heat and bring down.

4. Cover with a lid and keep overnight or for twenty-four hours to develop flavor.

Nutritional Information

27 calories 0g trans fat 2 mg sodium

0g protein 0 mg cholesterol 27 mg potassium

1g total fat 4g carbohydrate 18 mg phosphorus

0g saturated fat 0g fiber 9 mg calcium

Spicy Barbecue Sauce

Ingredients

¼ cup of dark corn syrup

¼ cup of red wine vinegar

¼ cup of onion, chopped

1 cup of water

2 teaspoons dry mustard

1 teaspoon Tabasco® pepper sauce

2 tablespoons olive oil

1 tablespoon all-purpose flour

1 teaspoon Mrs. Dash® (of your choice)

Preparations

1. Combine all ingredients in a cooking pan except olive oil and flour.

2. Mix olive oil and flour together in a separate bowl. Make into a paste.

3. Combine the paste with other ingredients in the saucepan, cook on low heat until it thickens

4. Add unto grilled or baked meat

Nutritional Information

28 calories 0g trans fat 28 mg sodium

0g protein 0 mg cholesterol 34 mg potassium

1g total fat 2g carbohydrate 7 mg phosphorus

0g saturated fat 0g fiber 2 mg calcium

Baked Egg Custard

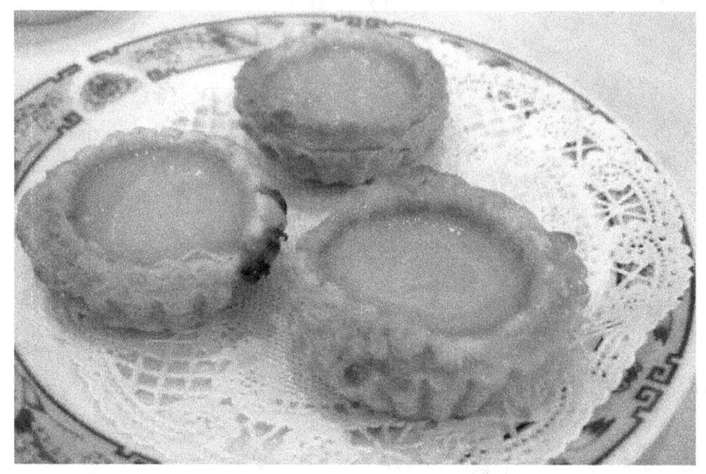

Ingredients

2 medium eggs

¼ cup of 2% milk

3 tablespoons stevia

1 teaspoon vanilla or lemon extract

1 teaspoon nutmeg

Preparations

1. Preheat oven to 325°F.

2. Combine all ingredients, and beat for one minute with an electric mixer until thoroughly mixed.

3. Pour into custard cups or muffin pans.

4. Sprinkle some nutmeg on it.

5. Bake for about 20-30 minutes. Watch how the knife comes out clean.

Nutritional Information

70 calories 0g trans fat 34 mg sodium

3g protein 91 mg cholesterol 30 mg potassium

3g fat 9g carbohydrate 42 mg phosphorus

1 saturated fat 0g fiber 12 mg calcium

Pineapple Pudding

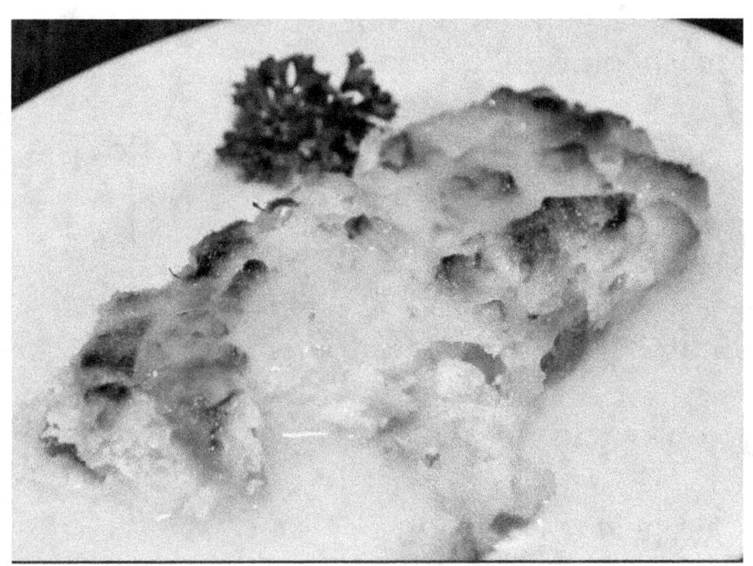

Ingredients

3 tablespoons all-purpose flour

½ cup of custard

1 large egg, whole

3 large eggs, divided

1 cup of 2% milk

1 cup of water

1 teaspoon vanilla extract

2 cups of pineapple chunks, drained

¼ cup of stevia powder

25-30 vanilla wafers

Preparations

1. Preheat oven to 425°F.

2. Combine flour, stevia, 1 whole egg and 3 egg yolks in top of a double boiler.

3. Add milk and water. Cook, uncovered over boiling water, stir until it thickens.

4. Bring down from the heat, and add vanilla extract.

5. Spread a small amount of the custard on the bottom of a 1 ½ quart casserole dish; top with half of the vanilla wafers, and half of the pineapple.

6. Keep on with layers of custard, vanilla, wafers, and pineapple, beginning and ending with custard.

7. Beat remaining egg whites with a hand mixer, add stevia. Beat until stiff peaks form.

8. Pour the egg whites on top of the layered pudding. Bake for 5 minutes or until lightly browned.

Yield: 12

Nutritional Information

209 calories 0g trans fat 80 mg sodium

4g protein 81 mg cholesterol 120 mg potassium

5g total fat 38g carbohydrate 71 mg phosphorus

2g saturated fat 1gram fiber 47 mg calcium

Lemon Crispies

Ingredients

1 cup of unsalted butter or margarine

1 cup of stevia powder

1 egg

1 ½ teaspoons lemon extract

1 ½ cup of all-purpose flour, sifted

Preparations

1. Preheat oven to 375°F.

2. Add and combine butter and stevia.

3. Combine your egg and lemon extract, whisk until light and fluffy.

4. Pour in the flour, mix until smooth.

5. Drop the butter by level tablespoon onto an ungreased cookie sheet, at least 2" apart.

6. Bake for about 10 minutes till color changes to brown

7. Take away from cookie sheet after letting it cool.

Nutritional Information

115 calories 0g trans-fat 12 mg sodium

2gram protein 76 mg cholesterol 20 mg potassium

6g total fat 12g carbohydrate 23 mg phosphorus

1gram saturated fat 0g fiber 7 mg calcium

Yield: 5

Spritz Cookies

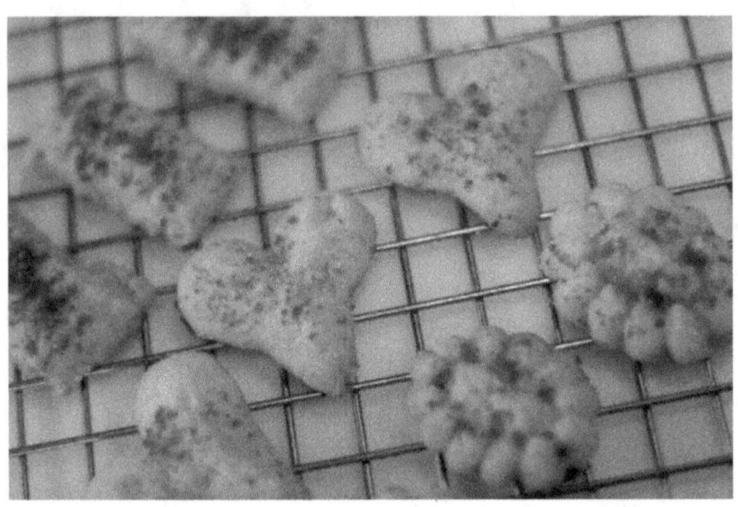

Ingredients

5 cups of all-purpose flour

2 cups of butter plus 2 tablespoons stevia powder

2 eggs

1 teaspoon almond extract

2 teaspoons vanilla extract

Preparations

1. Preheat oven to 400°F.

2. Combine flour, butter and stevia.

3. Add eggs and extracts; mix with a spoon or hand mixer on low speed.

4. Transfer cookies to a baking sheet

5. Bake for 5-8 minutes.

6. Allow to cool then serve when done

Nutritional Information

109 calories 0g trans fat 44 mg sodium

1gram protein 10 mg cholesterol 15 mg potassium

5g total fat 14g carbohydrate 10 mg phosphorus

3g saturated fat 0g fiber 7 mg calcium

Cream Cheese Cookies

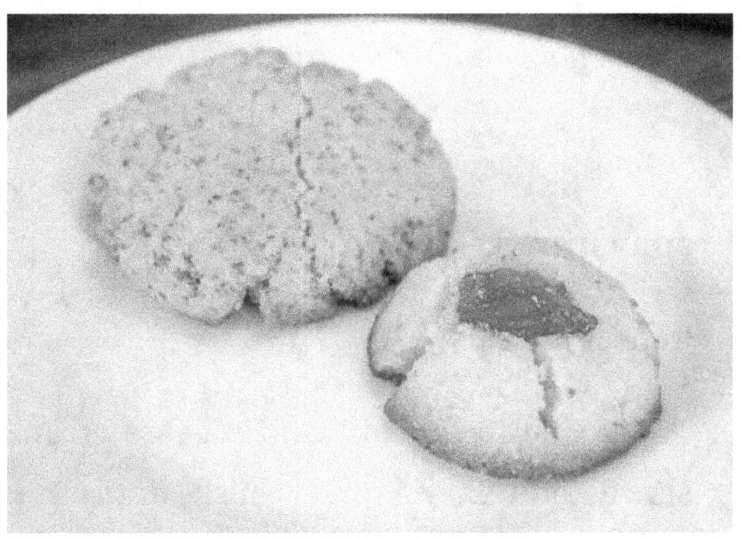

Ingredients

1 cup of butter or margarine, softened

1 3-ounce package cream cheese, softened

1 cup of stevia

1 egg yolk

2 ½ cups of all-purpose flour

1 teaspoon vanilla extract

candied cherry halves

Preparations

1. Preheat oven to 325°F.

2. Make butter-cream and cheese-cream; slowly add stevia and whisk until it is fluffy.

3. Add egg yolk; mix with flour and vanilla,

4. Keep in the freezer for at least 1 hour

5. Make the dough into a cookie and set on baking sheet

6. Gently press a cherry half into each cookie.

7. Bake for about 12-15 minutes.

Nutritional Information

80 calories 0g trans fat 31 mg sodium

0.5g protein 13 mg cholesterol 15 mg potassium

4g total fat 11g carbohydrate 14 mg phosphorus

2g saturated fat 0g fiber 6 mg calcium

Pineapple Pound Cake

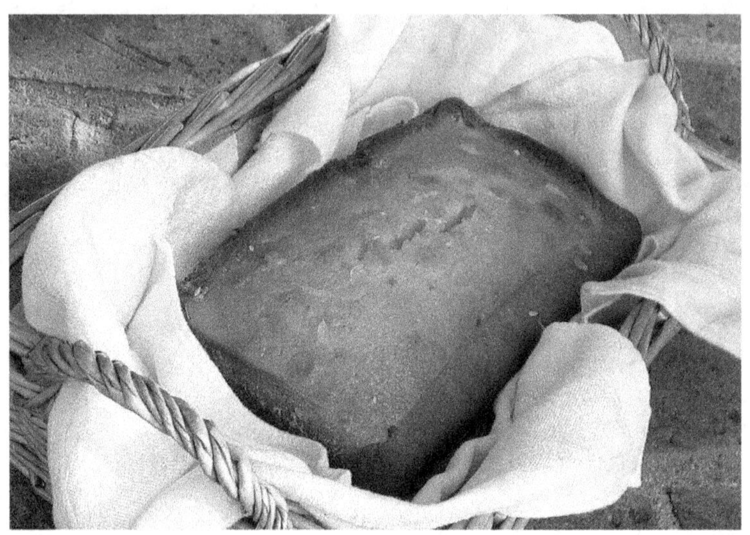

Ingredients for cake

3 cups of stevia

1 ½ cups of butter

6 whole eggs and 4 egg whites

1 teaspoon vanilla extract

3 cups of all-purpose flour, sifted

1 10-ounce can crushed pineapple (drain and reserve juice)

Preparations

1. Preheat oven to 350°F.

2. Combine stevia and butter and mix until smoothly mixed.

3. Add double eggs and mix with it.

4 Add vanilla with your flour and mix.

5. Put your drained, crushed pineapple And Bake between 45 minutes to 1 hour.

7. In a medium saucepan, mix together ingredients and stir.

8 Boil and remove when done. Pour over the cake

Nutritional Information

288 calories 0g trans-fat 93 mg sodium

2.5g protein 68 mg cholesterol 67 mg potassium

9g total fat 47g carbohydrate 47 mg phosphorus

6g saturated fat 19g fiber 19 mg calcium

Fruit in the Clouds

Ingredients

1 can fruit cocktail, drained

1 can apple juice, drained

8 ounces whipped cream, frozen

Preparations

1. Combine and mix all ingredients together.

2. Keep in a refrigerator.

Nutritional Information

113 calories 0g trans fat 20 mg sodium

1gram protein 0 mg cholesterol 152 mg potassium

3g total fat 23g carbohydrates 29 mg phosphorus

2g saturated fat 2g fiber 24 mg calcium

Fruit Salad

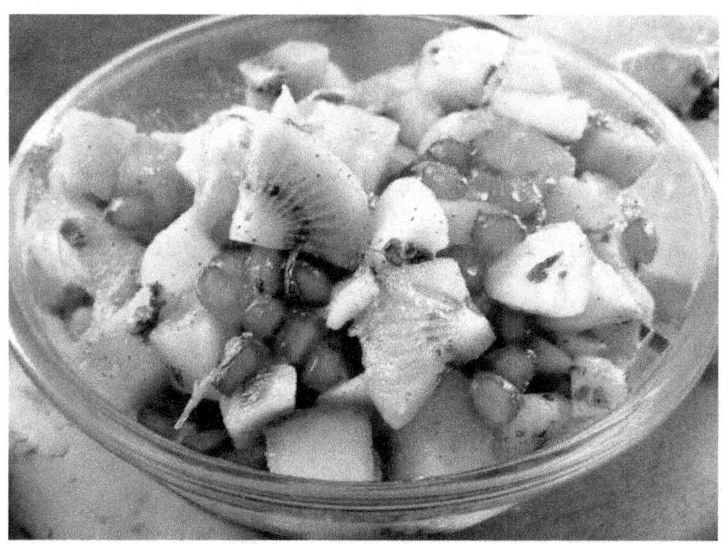

Ingredients

2 cups of canned fruit cocktail, drained

1 cup of canned pineapple chunks, drained

1 cup of whole or sliced strawberries, hulled

1 cup of apple, peeled, cored and diced

1 cup of marshmallows

½ cup of non-dairy whipped topping

Preparations

1. Combine all fruits in a big bowl.

2. Add marshmallows and whipped topping; mix well.

3. Refrigerate and serve when ready.

Nutritional Information

57 calories 0g trans fat 9 mg sodium

1g protein 0 mg cholesterol 120 mg potassium

0g total fat 14g carbohydrates 15 mg phosphorus

0g saturated fat 1gram fiber 14 mg calcium

APPENDIX

Frequently Asked Questions (FAQ)

How Much Alcohol Is Safe?

Consult your doctor to find out what's good for you.

Should Persons With Kidney Disease Need A Fluid Restriction?

A fluid restriction should be started when it's one of the recommendations given by your doctor. Do not begin a limited fluid program unless you have confirmation from your health care providers first.

How Can I Tell If My Food Is High Or Low In Potassium?

Almost all foods contain potassium. The fact that one product lists potassium and a similar product doesn't does not mean the similar product contains zero potassium. For instance, another brand of apple juice may not list potassium in the Nutrition Facts table at all, whereas one brand of apple juice may list 200 mg potassium in ¾ cup of juice. Though both brands of apple juice may contain about 200 mg potassium in ¾ cup, the labeling laws do not mandate that potassium content be listed.

What do the numbers of potassium content in a Nutrition Facts table mean? When deciding if a food has a lot or a little potassium use the following guidelines (however, always check with your renal dietitian for personal guidelines):

- Very low potassium: less than 40 mg per serving (1 %)

- Low potassium: less than 100 mg per serving (3%)

- Medium potassium: 100-250 mg per serving (3-7%)

- High potassium: 250-500 mg per serving (7-14%)

- Very high potassium: more than 500 mg per serving (>14%)

Do I Need To Take Mineral And Vitamin Supplements?

Vitamins and minerals are the essential chemicals and nutrients that the body needs for optimal development. People with chronic kidney disease (CKD) those who have chronic dialysis will not be so fortunate since they may be undergoing one form of diet limitation because of the kidney dialysis they are going through. These patients need water-soluble vitamins like vitamin B. Again; there is adequate need to avoid a general build-up of ions in the body. The fat-soluble vitamins like K, E and A and minerals such as phosphorus and potassium should not be replaced unless otherwise stated by your physician.

A very popular disease condition of the kidney is called kidney stones, or bladder stones. Recently it was noticed that phytochemicals such as catechin, epicatechin, epigallocatechin-3-gallate, diosmin, rutin, quercetin, hyperoxide, and curcumin were good sources of antioxidants and found to be good choices in preventing the development of bladder stones. These plant products have properties that include a diuretic, antispasmodic, and antioxidant capabilities.

Plus, they can inhibit the crystallization and clumping of crystals. Another recent article suggested that people with recurrent kidney stones should keep their dietary calcium intake in normal ranges so that the potential for increased urinary oxalate excretion can be avoided. Some of the existing literature on dietary approaches to preventing kidney disease include suggestions such as increasing fluids, limiting sodium, consuming citrates, keeping protein consumption moderate and increasing fruits and vegetables.

Menu Plan

Day 1

Breakfast

Oven fried chicken (*see ingredients in section 3.0 above*)

8 ounces Skim Milk

Lunch

Chili Rice with Beef (*see ingredients in section 3.0 above*)

Fresh peach

Water

Dinner

Swedish Meatballs (*see ingredients in section 3.0 above*)

Water

Nutritional information: *see details in section above*

Day 2

Breakfast

Steak and Onion Sandwich (*see ingredients in section 3.0 above*)

8 ounces Skim Milk

Lunch

Taco Stuffing (*see ingredients in section 3.0 above*)

Apple juice

Water

Dinner

Chicken Salad Delight (*see ingredients in section 3.0 above*)

Water

Nutritional information: *see details in section above*

Day 3

Breakfast

Seafood Croquettes (*see ingredients in section 3.0 above*)

8 ounces Skim Milk

Lunch

Chicken and rice (*see ingredients in section 3.0 above*)

Strawberry juice

Water

Dinner

Baked Fish (*see ingredients in section 3.0 above*)

Water

Nutritional information: *see details in section above*

Day 4

Breakfast

Crab cakes (*see ingredients in section 3.0 above*)

Cranberry juice

Water

Lunch

Turkey Barbecue Cups (*see ingredients in section 3.0 above*)

Grapefruit juice

Water

Dinner

Shrimp salad (*see ingredients in section 3.0 above*)

Water

Nutritional information: *see details in section above*

Day 5

Breakfast

Salisbury Steak (*see ingredients in section 3.0 above*)

8 ounces Skim Milk

Water

Lunch

Fish Tacos (see ingredients in the section above)

Fresh peach

Water

Dinner

Seafood Supreme (*see ingredients in the section above*)

Water

Nutritional information: *see details in section above*

Day 6

Breakfast

Lemon Chicken (*see ingredients in section 3.0 above*)

Strawberry juice

Water

Lunch

Turkey and Noodles (*see ingredients in section 3.0 above*)

Cranberry juice

Water

Dinner

Basic Meat Loaf (*see ingredients in section 3.0 above*)

Water

Nutritional information: *see details in section above*

Day 7

Breakfast

Corn Pudding (*see ingredients in section 3.0 above*)

8 ounces Skim Milk

Water

Lunch

Stuffed green Peppers (*see ingredients in section 3.0 above*)

Apple juice

Water

Dinner

Herbed Omelet (*see ingredients in section 3.0 above*)

Water

Nutritional information: *see details in section above*